BRINGING COMPUTERS TO THE HOSPITAL BEDSIDE

AN EMERGING TECHNOLOGY

Springer Publishing Company, Inc.
536 Broadway
New York, NY 10012

90 91 92 93 94 / 5 4 3 2 1

Library of Congress Cataloging-in-Publication Data

Bringing computers to the hospital bedside : an emerging technology /
    editors, Patrick F. Abrami and Joyce E. Johnson.
        p.   cm.
    Includes bibliographical references.
    ISBN 0-8261-7190-7
    1. Hospital care—Data processing.   2. Medical care—Data
processing.   3. Patient monitoring—Data processing.   I. Abrami,
Patrick F.   II. Johnson, Joyce E.
    [DNLM: 1. Computers.   2. Hospital Information Systems.   3. Medical
    Records.   WX 26.5 B858]
RA972.B65   1990
362.1′1′0285—dc 20
DNLM/DLC
for Library of Congress   90-9456
                                                                              CIP

Printed in the United States of America

Contents

Foreword

The challenge words for health care delivery in the 1990s are cost effectiveness, quality, and access. The front line of the escalation in the battle to provide patient care and contain costs will be the acute care hospital. To successfully meet the challenge will require harnessing the emerging technologies, especially those in information systems. But how? Equally important is *which* emerging technology to grasp onto, particularly when the implementation will cost millions of scarce dollars. These decisions will be made in an environment where future technology can make these investments obsolete before the full pay back of costs is made and benefits are realized.

In *Bringing Computers to the Hospital Bedside: An Emerging Technology*, co-editors Patrick F. Abrami and Joyce E. Johnson and the chapter authors identify the important issues surrounding the most exciting of the emerging technologies—bedside computer terminals. Bedside computing is such a natural extension of information systems technology. It provides the potential for faster, more accurate transmission of clinical and financial data. It also provides the means for better patient care and clinical decisionmaking.

Topics include the industry state of the art, conducting of cost-benefit studies before and after implementation, and practical points from hospitals that have worked with this technology. As working professionals, the book's authors bring the practical side of the issues involved in this technology to life. This is possible because they have spent the past two years working with it.

The editors and authors got to know each other, and the topic, through the Applied Management Systems and New England Healthcare Assembly seminars dedicated to bedside computer terminals held in Boston, San Francisco, and Dallas. The enthusiastic response of over 600 people who attended the seminars was a motivating force for the book.

So this book was really two years in the making and constitutes a most authorative first text in this important area. Enjoy it!

Alan J. Goldberg
President
Applied Management Systems, Inc.
Burlington, MA

Introduction

The bedside computer terminal concept, sometimes referred to as the point-of-care terminal concept, is the logical next step in the expansion of computer technology in hospitals today. Prior to this period, systems that provided clinical data were only extended to the nursing station, not into the patient's room.

Computer automation has evolved in hospitals since the early 1960s. In those early years, systems were focused primarily on financial applications such as general ledger and patient billing. Larger hospitals experimented with self-developed clinical systems, most of which failed. Clinical applications in most hospitals were not even considered seriously during this period. Remember that hardware was large and expensive in those days.

However, by the end of the 1960s, many companies were founded that provided computer support for financial applications on a shared basis. This approach was prevalent throughout most of the 1970s. By the mid-1970s, the first commercially offered order communication system (order entry) systems began to appear. This was a first step to bringing computer terminals to the nursing station and to ancillary departments. The one exception during the early 1970s was the emergence of Technicon, which offered a system that not only did order communication, but automated nurse charting and other nursing functions. This was a very expensive system and, generally, embraced only by large hospitals.

During the late 1970s and early 1980s, when hardware costs began coming down, it became possible to place computers in many departments. There was the emergence of many computer software companies that began specializing in departmental systems in such areas as laboratory, radiology, and pharmacy. Many of these systems were linked to the order communication system through interfaces. Many hospitals began to receive results at the nursing station through these interfaces.

The 1980s saw an explosion of computer technology availability for all size hospitals. Many new computer software companies that specialized in hospital software emerged during this period. These companies offered turnkey solutions to many small and medium hospitals. Many of these hospitals moved away from the shared concept to one in which turnkey software was placed on hardware based in the hospital. In today's environment, it is not unrealistic for hospitals of any size to have all financial systems, order entry, results reporting, departmental systems, and, to a certain degree, nursing functions automated. The reality is that the technology exists and that not every hospital has automated to this degree as yet, although many are moving in this direction.

Bedside technology simply extends the functionality that exists in many clinical nursing-station-oriented systems to the bedside. The rationale for this is simply that the patient is located there. With this type of approach taken to its farthest, all clinical and other data about the patient can be entered as it is being gathered, and data and clinical results from other departments can be accessible in the room with the patient. The proponents of this approach are saying that this can lead to a nearly paperless medical record. Many are already talking about a future that will see systems interacted with via voice recognition.

This step, which has already begun, is a long one. Hospitals and risk-taking vendors first began developing bedside systems in the mid-1980s. As Erica Drazen explains in Chapter 1 of this book, the bedside computer terminal concept really represents a broad class of systems, each with its own levels of integration, degree of functionality, and usefulness to health-care providers. She provides information about who is actually utilizing the concept today. The surprising conclusion is that not many hospitals have made the decision to venture into these uncharted waters.

Patrick Abrami, who researched Chapter 2, thought real-life experiences would be of interest to those reading this book. Therefore, the second chapter deals with actual case studies of six hospitals that have decided to be pioneers. Healthcare professionals at these six hospitals completed questionnaires about their bedside computer implementation. Topics covered include a chronology of implementation events, how the system was justified, benefits derived, implementation problems, where the terminals are actually located, interfaces to other hospital systems, and perceptions of those using the system. The names of these hospitals were shielded to insure against breach of confidentiality.

This book is not designed to be very technical in nature. However, in Chapter 3, we thought it would be helpful for those not technically oriented to gain some insight into some of the technical requirements of systems such as these. Robert Cort and Albert Crawford of the Graduate Health System developed a straightforward review of some technical considerations. Their remarks are accented by real-life experiences with the implementation of a fully integrated bedside terminal system at the Graduate Hospital, Philadelphia, PA.

In Chapter 4, there is a shift from technical to practical considerations. Patricia McNeal addresses some of the real, not-to-be-overlooked issues surrounding the concept. She also addresses some of the legal issues that are present, as well as patient confidentiality questions.

Chapter 5, written by Arthur St. Andre and Susan Eckert, focuses on the intensive care unit (ICU) bedside concept. This is one of the many varieties of systems that fall within this class of systems. As will be seen, the focus of these systems is to interface many monitoring devices to the bedside computer—that is, from patient directly to computer. This differs significantly from most of the other systems being discussed in this book. Therefore, it was decided to dedicate a chapter strictly to the concept.

Joyce Johnson wrote Chapter 6 of this book. She presents findings from a survey of nonusers of the concept about their perceptions, both positive and negative. These results were from a survey jointly prepared and conducted by Applied Management Systems, Inc., Burlington, MA and the Washington Hospital Center, Washington, D.C. The survey was of nurses and physicians only. The results are extremely positive.

All who have ventured into a major computer system conversion or implementation are aware that it is not easy. Much time, energy, coordination, and thought must go into the effort. This is especially true with the bedside concept and the types of functions that are automated. These systems require changes within the heart of what has been traditional care delivery for decades. Frances Vlasses discusses these issues and provider strategies for easing the strain caused by deep-seated change within Chapter 7. She reminds us that an organization's unique identity is carefully imprinted in the work setting. This must be understood if change is to be successful.

Although not many hospitals have embraced the concept as yet, many are evaluating whether to move in this direction. The suggestions and findings in Chapter 8, written by Louis Freund, will be helpful in any hospital's evaluation of the cost/benefit of moving forward. He discusses how to design a benefits evaluation and the results of three actual studies that he conducted for MECON.

The final chapter, Chapter 9, is a response to the Secretary's Commission on Nursing report in which computer technology and, specifically, bedside computer technology are mentioned as solutions to the shortage of nurses. This chapter, compiled by Mark Gross, Joyce Johnson, and Lillian Gibbons, also takes a look forward as to how this technology can play a major role in increasing nursing productivity and quality in the hospital setting.

This book is designed to fill a void on current facts about the concept. The editors, Patrick Abrami and Joyce Johnson, both feel that even more comprehensive materials will come forth on this topic as it evolves and matures. Thanks is extended to all the authors who took time to contribute their knowledge to this first-of-a-kind book.

Contributors

Arthur C. St. Andre, M.D., is clinical director of surgical critical care services at the Washington Hospital Center, Washington, D.C. He is a board certified intensivist and critical care physician who has been quite interested in clinical database management in the intensive care unit setting. He developed an interest in computing as a programmer in high school and, in recent years, his efforts have been directed toward effective utilization and development of a CDMS within the surgical intensive care units at the Washington Hospital Center. He received his B.S. at the University of Notre Dame and his M.D. from Thomas Jefferson Medical College.

Robert Cort, M.B.A., is the Director of Information Services at the Graduate Health System in Philadelphia, Pennsylvania. One of his responsibilities has been the installation of an integrated bedside patient care system at the Graduate Hospital. Mr. Cort is a strong advocate of integrated bedside patient care systems, and has made numerous presentations to various groups and organizations around the country discussing the implications of installing these systems. He holds an MBA from the Wharton School of Business and a Bachelor of Science from Brown University.

Albert G. Crawford, M.B.A., Ph.D., combines education and experience in teaching, research, health administration, and computer systems analysis and programming in his work as a systems analyst in the Department of Information Services of the Graduate Health System. As an analyst, he shares responsibility for implementation of the Health Data Sciences Ulticare Hospital Information System at

Graduate and has primary responsibility for research on that implementation. Dr. Crawford also specializes in providing computing support for clinical research at Graduate. He has recently collaborated in the development of two major research projects on disability among persons with AIDS. He has an MBA from Widener University and a Ph.D. from the University of Pennsylvania. He has held faculty positions at Widener University, Rutgers University, and Saint Joseph's University.

Erica L. Drazen, M.S., is a corporate Vice President and director of Arthur D. Little's Management Consulting Directorate. For the past 20 years, she has been involved in the evaluation of technology and services in medical care; her primary area of expertise is in the application of new technologies to improve health-care delivery. Currently, she manages a $5 million, 5-year program to plan for and successfully implement a comprehensive, integrated clinical computer system in Department of Defense hospitals, and maintains a research data base on bedside systems to support nursing care delivery and physician use of medical computers. Mrs. Drazen holds bachelor's and master's degrees in engineering from the Massachusetts Institute of Technology and is currently pursuing a doctorate in Health Policy and Management at Harvard School of Public Health.

Susan K. Eckert, M.S.N., is a specialist/surgical critical care nurse at the Washington Hospital Center, Washington, D.C. She has been actively involved with the bedside computer automation within the critical care areas at the Center. Prior to her joining the staff in Washington, she held positions at the Tulane University Hospital and the Massachusetts General Hospital. Ms. Eckert received her B.S.N. from Georgetown University and M.S.N. from Catholic University.

Louis E. Freund, Ph.D., has worked in health-care systems analysis and design for over 20 years. He joined the Industrial and Systems Engineering Department at San Jose State University, as an associate professor in the Fall of 1986, and is teaching in the areas of simulation, work measurement, engineering economics and statistics. During this period, he also became a senior consultant with MECON, where he has been responsible for designing and conducting studies that evaluate management systems and new technologies, that impact both the quality and quantity of services provided in health-care organizations. It is with MECON that he had the opportunity to conduct benefit studies of bedside computer systems.

Lillian K. Gibbons, M.P.H., Dr.P.H., is currently special assistant to the director of the NIH National Center for Nursing Research. As executive director of the Secretary's Commission on Nursing, U.S. Department of Health and Human Services, she recognized the importance of computer technology as an aid to the nurse of the future. Other recent positions were held at the Health Systems Division of Westinghouse Electric Corporation, a Congressional Fellow for the U.S. Senate Finance Committee, and regional advisor for the Pan American Health Organization and World Health Organization. She has a B.S. from Adelphi University School of Nursing, an M.P.H. from the University of Michigan School of Public Health, and Dr.P.H. from The Johns Hopkins University School of Hygiene and Public Health.

Mark S. Gross, B.S., is a partner in charge of Health Care Information Services Consulting for Ernst & Young. He has a B.S. degree in Biology from Farleigh Dickinson University in New Jersey. He has more than 20 years' experience in the health-care industry specializing in the information systems area, principally in planning, marketing and implementation of health-care systems. Prior experience includes the position of vice president, Information Services Group for Baxter Travenol, Inc., and 15 years' experience with IBM, having started as a marketing representative in 1968 in IBM's Washington, D.C. branch office after his discharge from active duty with the United States Air Force. His many years in the industry gives him a solid perspective on the growth of bedside computer technology.

Patricia McNeal, R.N., M.S.N., J.D., is an associate in the Philadelphia-based law firm of Sprecher, Felix, Visco, Hutchison & Young. As a professional consultant, she has provided expert case analysis for numerous hospitals in health law and medical malpractice cases, as well as medical peer review, risk management and quality assurance counsel to Philadelphia area hospitals. McNeal received her doctorate in jurisprudence from Temple University School of Law in 1989, earned a master's degree in health administration from Gwynedd

Mercy College, and received a bachelor of science degree in community health education from St. Joseph's University. McNeal earned a professional nursing diploma from Scranton's Community Medical Center School of Nursing. While at Graduate Hospital, she was actively involved with the implementation of the HDS bedside computer system.

Frances R. Vlasses, R.N., M.S.N., held a position for 4 years at the Graduate Hospital in Philadelphia, Pennsylvania, where she was directly involved with the implementation of the HDS bedside computer system. Her role was to develop and direct database development, training, and implementation approaches for the department of nursing. Prior to her involvement at the Graduate Hospital, she held positions at the Helene Fuld School of Nursing and Thomas Jefferson University Hospital. She is currently a consultant living in the Chicago area. She has taught at Widener University, Helene Fuld School of Nursing, University of Delaware, and Jefferson Medical College. She is a frequent speaker on numerous nursing topics including how to organize nurse staff for bedside documentation on an automated system. Vlasses received her B.S.N. from Villanova University and the M.S.N. from the Ohio State University.

1

Bedside Computer Systems Overview

Erica Drazen

The systems discussed in this book all have one thing in common: The presence of a computer terminal for data entry and retrieval in close proximity to the patient's bed. This step in the expansion of computer use in hospitals is very logical and, some would say, inevitable. Many other industries long ago discovered the benefits of capturing information at the point-of-service. The viewpoints on how best to structure and integrate these systems with a hospital-wide information system varies considerably, and each system on today's market takes a different tact. And these computer devices cover a broad range of hardware sophistication.

This chapter contains a discussion of the current status of bedside terminal systems from two perspectives: The types of systems that are being developed and marketed, and the reactions of early system users. It is important to note that this is an emerging technology. Most of the products are evolving quite rapidly, and the experiences of the early users have identified issues that are actively being worked on by users and vendors. Therefore, the chronological context of our observations is important; the state of the art will likely change in six–twelve months.

The information for this discussion comes from the following sources: an industry database maintained by Arthur D. Little, a survey that we conducted among users in December of 1988, and discussions with users and vendors conducted at conferences on bedside systems. The vendor database includes information on bedside systems since they were first introduced into the commercial marketplace or, for the earliest vendors, since February 1987. The vendor database now contains information on the features offered, the technical characteristics, the cost, and the installed base of fifteen vendors. This database is compiled using a semiannual telephone survey supplemented by site visits to the vendors.

The user database contains survey information on use of system features, satisfaction, benefits, and suggestions for improvements from 200 nurses who are direct users of three different bedside system products based in nine different acute care hospitals. The user database has been supplemented by visits to user sites, where we observed systems in use and conducted interviews with users.

DEFINITION OF BEDSIDE SYSTEM

The definition of a bedside data entry system has evolved with the development of the products and markets. Bedside data entry is a subset of a larger category of products involving data entry at the point of encounter. To qualify as a bedside system, a product must allow data entry and retrieval in an inpatient room and support documentation of a primary patient encounter. (Most current systems are used primarily to support nursing.) A bedside nursing system will, at a minimum, support retrieval of test results, entry of nursing care plans and orders, and documentation of the nursing care delivery process. Many of the systems on the market do go beyond this minimum use requirement.

Currently, three different types of products meet most of the above criteria:

- Dedicated products for general medical/surgical care
- Dedicated products for ICU/critical care
- Integrated hospital information systems that contain bedside data entry and retrieval

Although a year ago it appeared that these systems were quite different, the distinctions among products appears to be blurring. Systems originally implemented in general medical and surgical units are being tested in the ICU environment and stand-alone systems are being interfaced to hospital information systems (HIS). Despite these trends, we expect that these three categories of products will, in the long term, be sold into three separate markets with different competitors, buying criteria, and decision makers.

General Nursing Support Systems

The largest installed base of bedside systems is of the first type: systems dedicated to providing nursing support to general medical and surgical units.

The following three examples illustrate the range of bedside products being marketed to general medical and surgical units. Table 1.1 lists other companies in this marketplace.

- MedTake, a product offered by Micro Healthsystems, has the largest installed customer base. The MedTake product was intro-

Table 1.1. Vendors Offering Bedside Systems

Baxter/CliniCom
CliniCom Incorporated
Critikon
Health Data Sciences Inc.
HBO/CliniCom
Micro Healthsystems
Second Foundation, Inc.
SMS/CliniCom
SMS
TDS
3M HELP Patient Care System
*ACT-PC
*EMTEK
*Hewlett Packard
*Trinity
*Marquette

*Critical Care Systems-ICU

duced in 1986; in recent years, this system has consistently captured the largest number of new hospital installations and has expanded the number of beds in hospitals using its system. The MedTake product is designed to operate as a stand-alone, dedicated product for nursing support, though it can be interfaced to financial or ancillary systems. MedTake used a specially designed terminal with keys to access most functions. This makes the system very easy to learn and use.

- CliniCom is another of the early bedside system developers. Its system uses either a hand-held terminal, a wall-mounted touch screen, or both. The CliniCom product is dedicated to providing nursing support and is always interfaced to another vendor's HIS. The CliniCom systems in use today are interfaced to HIS products from Baxter, HBO, and SMS. CliniCom is the only vendor marketing a hand-held terminal.

- CritiKon introduced a bedside system for general medical and surgical units about 1 year ago. This product only operates as a standalone system. It accepts data from an electronic thermometer and noninvasive blood pressure cuff.

Most dedicated nursing systems for general medical and surgical unit support have, or are developing, capabilities to support functions such as nursing assessment, care planning, charting of care delivered, medication charting (with an interface to a pharmacy system), results reporting (with a laboratory system interface), and input and output calculations. Since these products are still evolving, the capabilities offered on each system vary widely. Some have only four or five capabilities operational; others have up to fifteen. Figure 1.1 shows the number of vendors offering different bedside capabilities.

In addition to the functions of the bedside system itself, systems vary in the level of integration or interfacing capability vary in the extent to which the interfaces have been actually implemented. One reason that few system interfaces are operational is that interfaces are expensive and, therefore, are usually not implemented when a system is being tested on a few units.

Other critical variables differ among systems as well. The ability to tailor the system to meet hospital needs, downtime experience, and ease of use are all important features to consider.

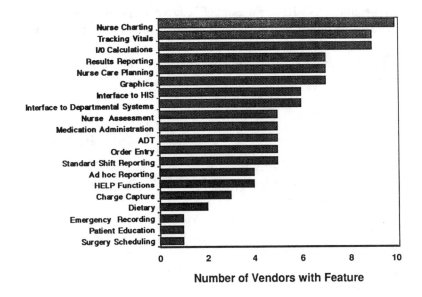

FIGURE 1.1. Availability of functions in systems for general medical and surgical care.

Some systems are so easy to use that they can be learned in a few hours, therefore making it feasible to train agency or float staff to use the system. Other systems are much more complex and difficult to learn. Such systems are likely to be successful only in units with stable, permanent staffing.

A system to support nursing care must be available whenever nursing care is delivered. This almost always translates to 24 hours per day, 7 days per week. A survey of early users indicated that this level of availability has not been achieved by all systems. Since failure is never totally avoidable, it is also important to ensure that when the system does go down that effective mechanisms exist to prevent data from being lost.

The ability to tailor the system is important for two reasons. To minimize the amount of change being introduced, each hospital will want to tailor the screens to match closely the format, content, and terminology of existing paper documents. Since the systems are still evolving, hospitals will want to have the ability to adapt screens for different purposes. If, for example, charting the number of visits happens to be important, a hospital might want to be able to adapt a screen designed for charting vital signs to record this information. Systems that can be easily modified and vendors that have mechanisms for sharing enhancements among users will have products that evolve faster and achieve higher levels of acceptance.

ICU Systems

Bedside systems for the ICU have been in the marketplace for a shorter period of time than general nursing support systems. These systems are designed to accept, analyze, and display data from monitoring equipment, support the same types of nursing functions as the systems for the general medical/surgical wards; and support the extensive flowcharting function and graphics requirements of the ICU. Uninterrupted performance and requirements for tailoring are even more stringent in the ICU environment. Most ICU systems also can provide data for both patient care and research. Although they are newer to the marketplace, ICU systems are gaining initial acceptance; and since the systems are more expensive, the total dollar investment in ICU bedside automation may quickly exceed that invested in acute care systems.

As seen in Table 1.1, EMTEK, Marquette, Trinity, and ACT PC have ICU systems installed now, and Hewlett Packard recently announced its entry into this marketplace. EMTEK currently has the largest base of bedside ICU systems installed.

Total Hospital Systems

The third type of bedside product is the total hospital information system that incorporates bedside data entry. These systems have the same support for nursing described earlier, plus they allow any functions on the hospital information system to be accessed from the bedside. Therefore, this type of bedside system is typically used for entry of orders, results reporting, review of results status, review of medications, etc. The total hospital systems with bedside access are often used by physicians as well as nurses since they provide easy access to patient information.

Health Data Sciences was the earliest, and perhaps the best known, example of an integrated HIS using bedside data entry. The HELP system from 3M is another system in this category. TDS has experimented with providing bedside data entry with its system, and SMS has developed and tested a system with new software designed for bedside support connected to its HIS.

DIFFUSION OF BEDSIDE COMPUTING

As seen in Table 1.1, a number of vendors are interested in this marketplace. That list has grown slightly over the last few years. Two firms have exited the business, but more have entered.

Figure 1.2 and 1.3 shows the growth in hospitals using bedside systems over the past 2 years, and Figure 1.4 and 1.5 shows the number

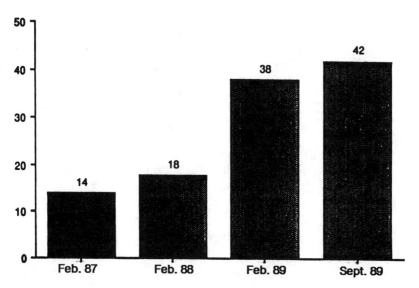

FIGURE 1.2. The hospital market is moving beyond beta testing: Hospitals using acute care systems.

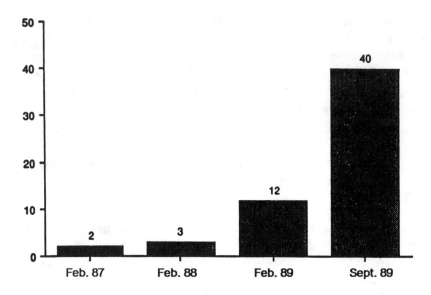

FIGURE 1.3. Penetration of critical care systems is still low: Hospitals with critical care systems.

of terminals that have been installed. These graphs illuminate several points. Although the growth in users has been continual, market penetration is still tiny. Less than 1% of bedsides in medium and large hospitals have computer support. The market is unstable; it is not large enough to support the number of vendors currently participating. Even with continued steady growth, we will likely see a shakeout of less financially stable or less committed companies.

Comparisons of the data within Figures 1.2–1.5 indicate that diffusion of bedsides within the hospitals has increased quite rapidly over the last few years. This is principally due to the fact that some hospitals tried out the dedicated nursing support systems on one or two wards and then made a decision to install bedside automation throughout the hospital.

The one question that is most frequently raised in discussions of bedside systems is, "Why have systems diffused so slowly?" Two years ago, one correct answer was that the market awareness about the product still needed to be developed. Certainly, we are now past that stage. Four to five well-attended conferences were held on

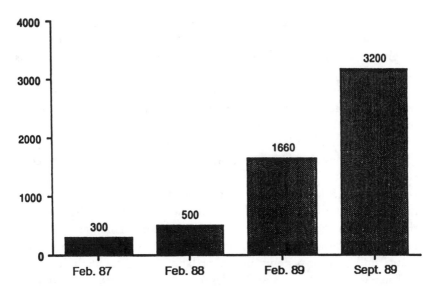

FIGURE 1.4. Growth of bedsides is accelerated by diffusion of terminals within the hospital: Terminals in general medical/surgical units.

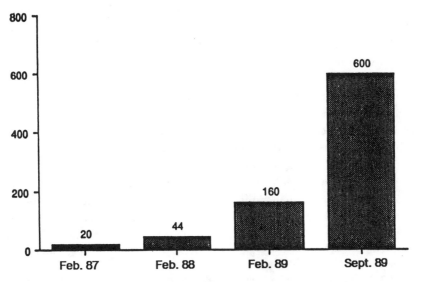

FIGURE 1.5. The number of terminals placed in critical care is growing quickly: Number of terminals in ICUs.

bedside systems last year; over 500 people attended these conferences; hundreds more were exposed to the technology through sessions at hospital meetings, articles, or direct sales. Although the technology is still evolving, today's products are useful in their current form, and users report high satisfaction and many benefits. Many products are available to choose from, and it does not appear that users are waiting for a technical breakthrough.

The motivation to buy bedside systems is also evident. Helping to solve the nursing problem is on every hospital chief executive officer's (CEO) priority list. Nurses who study bedside systems are widely convinced that they will provide real benefits, and one of the recommendations of the Secretary's Commission on Nursing Report was that "The Federal Government should sponsor further research and encourage health care delivery organizations to develop and use automated information systems and other labor saving technologies."*

The biggest barrier to system sales seems to be the cost of the systems and the financial constraints on the buyers. In a typical 250-bed hospital, the annual budget for HIS is about $600,000. The cost of the bedside systems for general medical and surgical care ranges from about $3,000 to about $10,000 per bed. ICU systems cost more than $20,000 per bed. When these numbers are multiplied by the number of bedsides to be automated, with the costs of maintenance and training included, and the total amortized over five years, a typical hospital would have to plan on a 50–100% increase in its information system expenditures.

This theoretical hospital will undoubtedly also receive cost offsets. A dramatic decline in end-of-shift overtime should occur when charting is done continuously. If nursing satisfaction increases, the cost of recruitment should go down because turnover will decrease. Improved documentation should also provide savings in time spent by nonnursing staff in accreditation, liability, and utilization review activities. Offsetting savings are more difficult to estimate than system costs, since they will vary greatly from site to site and few hospitals have published studies of their experience. Some of the early studies used inappropriate assumptions in converting time savings to

---

Source: Secretary's Commission on Nursing, Final Report. (December, 1988). Department of Health and Human Services, Office of the Secretary, Washington, D.C.

dollar benefits, which has made the available data less reliable. (A model for estimating and documenting dollar savings is presented in Chapter 8.) The diffusion of bedside systems is likely to continue to proceed slowly, with the prime drivers being the number of hospitals that can afford the capital expenditure and the skill of nursing and vendor staff in presenting their case for bedside support.

USER EXPERIENCE

In December 1988, Arthur D. Little conducted a survey of nurses in nine hospitals who were using three different bedside systems in general medical and surgical units. A total of 195 responses were received. To qualify for the study, a hospital had to be using the bedside system to replace paper documentation; and to meet the survey criteria, the nurse had to be using a bedside system to deliver patient care.

The majority of the respondents were registered nurses (RNs); they ranged in age from 18 to over 55. About half of the nurses had used a computer before, and almost 25% had taken a computer course.

The three products represented in the survey, CliniCom, Micro Healthsystems, and TDS, had, respectively, five, 12, and 15 functions in routine use. To adjust for this varying base, data on satisfaction with features are reported only for users who had experience with (were using) the feature. Nurses reported these system functions as very useful:

- Nursing assessment
- Nurse charting
- Tracking vital signs
- Intake/Output calculations
- Repiratory charting
- Medication charting
- Graphics
- Help functions

- Order entry
- Results reporting

Where they were available, nurses wanted to add the following:

- Order entry
- Nurse care planning
- Nurse charting
- Medication charting
- Documentation of patient education

There was consensus that the top three benefits gained from bedside systems were saved time in charting and documentation, improved documentation, and increased availability of patient information. There was a divergence of opinion about whether the bedside systems improved nursing satisfaction, nursing productivity, or quality of care.

The terminals being used were as important to satisfaction as the features offered. Systems with customized terminals were much more acceptable than systems using a standard terminal. One problem with the standard terminal was its size. Eighty percent of the nurses felt that the bedside device should be located on the wall. Most users expressed a preference for the type of device they were using; nurses using portable devices felt they were preferable, whereas nurses using stationary devices preferred this approach. Both groups agreed that having both stationary and portable devices available would provide them the best access. There was also consensus that devices should be available outside of the patient's room. Placement of the device within the room also is critical. Nurses do not like to turn their back to the patient to use the system. If devices are at a fixed height, they are difficult to use by short and tall staff. Also, the lighting on the screen was sometimes too bright to be used at night without disturbing the patient or too dim to light up the keyboard. These types of problems will undoubtedly be corrected in the next generation of bedside hardware.

Reliability of systems was not 100%. Users were asked how often in the last month the system was not available when they needed to use it. As can be seen in Figure 1.6, only about 25% of the nurses reported their system was never down. There are several reasons the system could have been unavailable. A new software upgrade could have been in process, the system could have been brought down for maintenance, or there could have been unplanned downtime. Whatever the cause, downtime must be reduced if these systems are being relied upon to support routine patient care.

Acceptance of the three different systems differed considerably. For one, only 36% of respondents felt that acceptance of the system by nurses was very high; for another system 60% reported high acceptance; and for the third system, 65% reported high acceptance. Almost all respondents reported high acceptance among patients. The acceptance and use of the bedside systems by physicians appeared to vary by hospital.

The survey results about acceptance among nurses reported satisfaction lower than in case studies. This may be because users respond

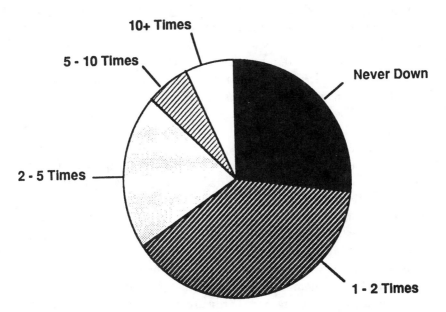

FIGURE 1.6. Reliability of systems: Number of times device wasn't available in last month.

differently in an anonymous survey, or it may be due to a difference in the interpretation of the words "acceptance" and "satisfaction."

The results of the user survey reflect on emerging technology environment. Users are tolerant of imperfections in their current system, yet have many suggestions for improvements. They see benefits in the systems they have installed, and most see the potential for enhanced benefits in the future.

Any users considering this technology need to recognize their pioneering role. The hospitals that get the most out of this technology will be those that simultaneously try to get benefits from current products and collaborate with vendors to develop improved products for the future.

FUTURE DEVELOPMENTS

The market for bedside systems is clear. It makes sense for the nurses to be able to provide and document care at the bedside, to eliminate redundant transcription, and to make records more complete, legible, and acceptable. The size of the market will depend on the number of hospitals that decide this is a priority investment. The market will grow more rapidly if federal or state money becomes available to fund technologies to address the nursing shortage, or if data can be productive that demonstrates clear cost savings, and if vendors and nursing staff develop successful approaches to marketing the systems to hospital decision makers.

The technology of bedside systems will continue to evolve. The hospital information systems business has traditionally been a software business. Most hardware has consisted of standard systems purchased from large computer vendors. One of the interesting facets of the bedside systems business is that hardware, especially the bedside terminal, is critical to success. Therefore, an opportunity exists to innovate and compete on the basis of both hardware and software. The rate of software evolution will depend on the investment made by the vendor and on the number of customers that participate in developing new applications. The rate of hardware development is almost entirely dependent on the level of investment by vendors. Because investment will be governed somewhat by sales, the evolution of the technology is also likely to proceed slowly.

External factors could also drive the market. The persistence of the nursing shortage and the types of staffing solutions developed may favor investment in bedside systems. Accreditation, reimbursement, or quality-of-care regulations impacting nursing could also create driving forces to automate at the bedside. The most likely bedside scenario involves development of two markets—one in the ICU and one in the other units—and slow but steady sales and product enhancement.

2

Six Case Studies

Patrick F. Abrami

This chapter outlines the experiences of six hospitals that have implemented and/or are still in the process of implementing the concept of bedside computer terminals. The case studies reflect the efforts in installing the Ulticare system offered by Heath Data Sciences, Inc. (HDS), the Medtake system offered by Micro Healthsystems, and the Clinicare system offered by CliniCom Incorporated. As has already been pointed out, these products are all designed to do differing things with a wide degree of functionality. The major common feature is that each utilizes some sort of input/output device in the patient's room. Although they do have some common functions, they diverge especially in their degree of integration with other systems. The hospitals implementing these systems all had one common trait: a willingness to be a pioneer in this new technology. They all experienced relatively long installation times and are still enhancing what they have done.

CASE SUMMARIES

Hospital A

Hospital A, a major teaching hospital on the east coast, was in need of a total revamping of their information system's strategy prior to their signing a contract with HDS in May of 1986. An aggressive administration and board decided to take a large leap forward and implement this fully integrated patient care information system with terminals at the bedside. This move was consistent with their existing decentralized charting which matched the Frieson-designed hospital. A *Frieson design* is one which minimizes the nursing station as the most important point on a nursing unit for all levels of communication about a patient. Instead, it stresses the importance of placing more of this communication at the bedside. This architectural philosophy is very similar to the information system philosophy of doing as much as possible in terms of data entry and retrieval at the bedside. Table 2.1 outlines the chronology of events.

This system was not cost justified per se. Since charts were already at the bedside, this approach fit nicely with an existing philosophy. Further, it was supported by the belief that the integration and scheduling would improve hospital efficiencies and thus decrease length of stay. Benefits to date have not yet been quantified; however, radiology reports are now available on time. The system also provides

Table 2.1. Hospital A Implementation Chronology

Date	Occurrence
May, 1986	Contract signed.
November, 1986	Registration/ADT implemented.
April, 1987	Rehabilitation Unit Implements Nursing, social work, OT, PT, and related physician orders.
	4S Cardiology Unit Implements similar functions.
January, 1988	Radiology system implemented.
December, 1988	Laboratory system implemented.
January, 1989	6N/6S—Surgery Units implemented.
	Nursing Admission Assessment, care plans, and shift assessments.
February, 1989	5N/5S—Medical Units—same as above
July, 1989	Order Entry (only lab, dietary, EEG, EKG).
September, 1989	ER order entry.
November, 1989	Radiology order entry.
November, 1989	Operating Room
January, 1990	Pharmacy system implementation.
March, 1990	Critical Case Unit implementation.

a positive environment for nursing to evaluate care planning and nursing diagnosis. There are possible benefits in the area of discharge planning and care planning, but studies are not yet complete.

Implementation problems include the pace of development by the vendor (since their product was still evolving); insufficient hospital staff to maintain the ever growing data base; quality assurance issues surrounding new releases or products that are caused by the pressure to get a product to market; problems in the amount of revisions needed to change work flow; chart management problems resulting from vast amounts of paper generated; and difficulties with badge readers, which must be utilized to let users sign onto the system. These problems are experienced by most initiators who choose to be among the first to implement a new and relatively untested product.

Terminals are currently located at nurse servers (pass-through closets between patient room and hallway). This was done after much input from staff regarding comfort and feasibility. Each terminal will be individually placed in ICU rooms. Adequate equipment did not exist to support wall or ceiling mounting at the bedside, which was preferable.

HDS is a fully integrated system. The other major systems which exist are the financials which are SMS product which did not integrate to HDS. Currently, nursing, physicians, and social workers utilize the system. The nursing clerical staff utilize the system to a certain degree. The nurses feel it is easy to learn, but not necessarily a time saver. They are still hoping for benefits from reduced telephone time for ordering tests/medications and receiving results, once the system is fully implemented. The physicians find the system easy to use, but too confining. Some physicians feel it is degrading to their profession, while others feel it is wonderful.

Hospital B

Hospital B, a community hospital located on the east coast, made a commitment to provide nurses an automated means of charting. Between September of 1987 and February of 1988, the hospital piloted the Micro Healthsystems Medtake system on B3, an acute medical/ surgical (M/S) unit. They were also an alpha test site for Medtake's new hardware. By October 1988, they signed a contract for the

Table 2.2. Hospital B Implementation Chronology

Date	Occurrence
November 1987	B3—acute Med/Surg trial commences
June 1988	4NA—Orthopedics/Neuro-Orthopedic enhancements
October 1988	Contract signed
November 1988	Installation of nursing care plan module
December 1988	Live A3 Oncology (oncology enhancements)
January 1989	Live 4NB—M/S
February 1989	Live 2W Telemetry (cardiac enhancements)
April 1989	Live 3N OB/GYN (OB/GYN enhancements)
April 1989	Installation of central processor (connecting units)
May 1989	Live Pediatrics (Peds enhancements)
May 1989	Nursing care plans live 4NA
July 1989	Live 4E—M/S
July 1989	Nursing care plans live A3 Oncology
September 1989	Live 3W—GU
December 1989	Live 3E—M/S
December 1989	Nursing care plans moved to additional units

implementation of the full Medtake system. Table 2.2 outlines the chronology of events. Note that "live" means that the personnel started utilizing the system in their daily routine.

The hospital cost justified this system through analysis which showed a savings in documentation time. Benefits realized to date include increased documentation quality, increased legibility, consistent use of terminology, all reports are up to date, and nursing care plans are now completed on a routine basis. It has also been quantified that documentation time has indeed decreased and there has been an elimination of overtime due to documentation.

Given that the system is not currently integrated to other major systems, the implementation went rather smoothly.

This hospital chose to locate their terminals at the base of the patient bed on a wall shelf. The terminals are securely bolted to the shelf. They found this location to be the most convenient and does not interfere with care.

The Medtake system is currently a stand-alone nursing system. The hospital utilizes Baxter financial systems and is planning to utilize the Baxter order entry system. Long-range plans call for integration to the Baxter systems. The hospital also utilizes the DecRad radiology system, Medlab laboratory system, and the Dose pharmacy system. Future plans also call for integration of Medtake with each of these systems. Currently, this system is predominantly utilized by nurses who feel it is easy to use and who feel it makes them more productive. Physicians can utilize the system for review purposes only. Some do because of the ease of use. Other professionals, such as social workers, physical therapy, and respiratory therapy also utilize the system for review purposes.

Hospital C

Hospital C, a rural community hospital located in New England, first became interested in bedside computer technology through its CEO. This interest spawned research into available systems during 1985. Nursing rejected a hand held product offered by NCR at the time. They felt the Ulticare system was too expensive for this size hospital. After further review, they selected the Medtake system. Negotiations began with Patient Care Technology (PCT), Medtake's parent company at the time. During the negotiation process and very near to the contract signing, PCT sold out to Micro Healthsystems, resulting in new talks and negotiations with the new company representatives. Final board approval was received in May 1986 and a contract was signed in July 1986. Table 2.3 outlines the chronology of events.

This system was justified by a belief that, with a shortage of RNs, it would make the lives of the remaining RNs easier. In addition, it was felt that overtime could be reduced. Benefits to date include documentation which is now always encoded with date, time, and initials, as well as a chart which, in general, has more information and a greater degree of accuracy. Quantitative benefits include an increase in productivity through the elimination of the need for manual data transcription, calculations and graphing, as well as by automating the entry of data into the chart. The amount of overtime was actually reduced.

Implementation went smoothly with the exception of hardware problems with its bedside terminals. After much research, Medtake finally identified a problem with one of the computer chips in the bedside unit. This chip was changed and they received all new bedside units and the problem was eliminated. Minor problems did occur with

Table 2.3. Hospital C Implementation Chronology

Date	Occurrence
July 1986	Contract signed
December 1986	System installation complete
January 1987	Employees trained
February 1987	All three nursing units came live (M/S, Obstetrical and ICU) with charting only.

the system over the next 6 months with company representatives traveling to Northern Vermont to rectify. The hospital was very happy with the excellent support given by their vendor during the first year.

Terminals were located between the beds in each room on special stands. This was the most convenient place for access by the nurse and close to an electrical outlet.

The version of Medtake implemented was an early product offering by Micro Healthsystems. Even though each of the three nursing units has a unit, each does not talk to the other. Patients are transferred by disc. The hospital has automated admission, discharge and transfer (ADT), patient accounting, general accounting, order entry, radiology, laboratory, and respiratory systems all on SMS software which is not integrated to the bedside software. The hospital has no plans for future integration. Currently, the nurses use and like the system very much. Due to cost reasons, the care planning and medication charting functions have been placed on hold. Occasionally, a physician will use the system to retrieve data, although most dislike the concept. No other professionals use the terminals.

Hospital D

Hospital D, a teaching hospital located on the west coast, was looking for a bedside solution which would involve their mainframe vendor, which was HBO running their STAR product. The decision was made to go with CliniCom and to initially interface the CliniCom system to the HBO ADT system and pharmacy system. During July and August 1988, contract negotiations were conducted with both vendors, resulting in agreements being reached by the end of August 1988. Table 2.4 outlines the chronology of events.

The hospital is hoping the pilot units will demonstrate that there will be an elimination/reduction of duplicate charting, improved productivity by having information easily accessible, and improved quality of care by reaching above goals and eliminating medication errors. The actual benefits will not be known until after the pilot studies have been completed.

Implementation problems included the orientation of staff to a keyboard which was different from the HIS. Since they were an alpha site for a new release of the software, it was difficult to keep up with the changing procedures and protocols. There were some hardware problems especially with transmission with the hand held devices. Physicians had a difficult time adjusting to the charge document changes. The live dates were changed four times due to software/integration problems.

Terminals are mounted on foot wall of each patient room. The project team reviewed nursing practice and determined this area would be the most accessible without intruding on the patient every time. Other installations had placed them in locations similar to their decision. The height recommended by Clinicom was agreed upon by nursing at the hospital.

As was mentioned, the hospital utilizes HBO-STAR software including ADT, patient accounting, general accounting, order entry, radiology, laboratory, pharmacy and respiratory applications. They are currently interfaced to ADT and pharmacy, and in some respects

Table 2.4. Hospital D Implementation Chronology

Date	Occurrence
August 1988	Contract signed
December 1988	Hardware installed on pilot units (2R-Respiratory and 5R-Orthopedic)
January 1989	Live on pilot units with V.S., fluids & weights
March 1989	Live with medication administration
July 1989	Results reporting at bedside
February 1990	Implementation of IV module
June 1990	Full implementation of all patient care units including ICU

interfaced to respiratory. Plans call for interfaces to patient accounting, order entry, as well as results reporting from laboratory and
radiology. The nurses currently use the system for V.S., fluids, and
weights. They find it fast to use and beneficial. Medication administration they find more difficult to use, since it is a major change in
practice. The physicians do not use the system as yet. This group is
upset with the change in their chart documents and formatting differences. Pharmacists also use the system. They feel that the use of bar
coding will save time in the pharmacy.

Hospital E

Hospital E, a teaching hospital located in the mid-west, was an early
user of the Medtake system. They started the process with a trial on
one nursing unit back in November 1985. In May 1986, a request for
proposal was sent to all available bedside terminal vendors offering
product at that time. By April 1987, a contract was signed with Micro
Healthsystems for the Medtake system. Table 2.5 outlines the chronology of events.

This system was justified on its perceived ability to save nurses time
and provide cost savings in reduced overtime. To date, the hospital
feels the system has been a real nurse satisfier. It enhances their ability
to recruit nurses, especially students who have used Medtake during
their clinical rotations. Medical Records personnel like the system
since documentation cannot get to them without patient identification
information. It has been quantified that overtime has actually been
reduced and that significant nurse time has been saved. A study is in
progress to formally document these savings. They have been able to
reduce their nursing worked hours per patient index because of the
efficiencies.

The hospital felt they had the normal software "glitches" when
major enhancements were made and that a lot of support was needed
to changing nursing behavior due to bedside charting. Overall the
implementation process was fairly smooth.

Most of the bedside terminals are located in the far corner of the
patient's room, on or near the foot wall. When this was not possible,
they put them in the safest, most utilitarian location they could find in
the room (in old clothes lockers, etc.).

Table 2.5. Hospital E Implementation Chronology

Date	Occurrence
April 1987	Contract signed
June 1987	6 West–OB/GYN began charting on original Medtake
July 1987	4 West–Telemetry unit began charting on original Medtake
September 1987	5 West–Surgical unit began charting on original Medtake
October 1987	6 East–Chronic unit and Med/Surg began charting on original Medtake
February 1988	Began development of a more sophisticated I and O application and graphic summary report
May 1988	Final approval of I and O applications
December 1988	Signed contract for Medtake 3000 product
December 1988	6 West/6 East—Install Medtake 3000
March 1988	4 West/5 West—Install Medtake 3000
April 1989	5 East/6 East—Install Medtake 3000
May 1989	4 East began charting on Medtake 3000
June 1989	Physical Rehab and Short Stay center began charting on Medtake 3000
July 1989	Cognitive Rehab charting on Medtake 3000
February 1989	Pediatrics charting on Medtake 3000
June 1990	Install in Peri-natal and ICU's, centralize Medtake, and develop Medtake/PCS interface
June 1991	Invite other care givers (RT, PT, etc.) to document on Medtake

Currently, Medtake is not interfaced to any other hospital system. The hospital utilizes the IBM-PCS ADT, patient accounting, order entry and respiratory systems, a VAX radiology system, a self developed laboratory system and the DOSE pharmacy system. At this juncture, there are plans to interface to the ADT, patient accounting and respiratory systems. Patient care staff (RNs, Licensed Practical Nurses (LPNs), Nurse's Aides (NAs) and clinical nurses) all perceive the system to be user friendly and valuable to them. Most attending physicians do not use the system. The only physicians using the system are medical students and residents for reviewing nursing documentation. Others who use the system for review purposes include nursing school faculty and students, as well as respiratory therapy, physical therapy, and dietary staff.

Hospital F

Hospital F, a teaching hospital located in the mid-west, started its search for bedside technology back in November 1986 when CliniCom first demonstrated their Clinicare product. In February 1987, the hospital signed a contract for a six week pilot study. During the next several months, studies were conducted. In June 1987, a contract was signed for a second pilot test, this time on the telemetry unit. They went live with the vital signs (VS) and fluid balance functions and eventually brought live medication administration. After complete review of the pilot study data, a house-wide contract with CliniCom was signed in April 1988. Table 2.6 outlines the chronology of events.

This system was justified through extensive pre- and post-studies during the pilot testing phase. A documented savings of 12 minutes per patient per day was removed from the existing patient classification system based on the studies. Qualitative benefits realized include more legible VS, fluid balance, and Medication Administration Record (MAR) reports, more timely medication administration, a decrease in medication errors, and a more timely medication dispensing from the pharmacy.

Implementation problems ranged from physician acceptance, to hardware reliability, to staff behavior changes with medication administration, and to the availability of hard copy data for clinicians. Overall, the implementation went as smoothly as expected.

The bedside terminals were located at the foot of the bed. The desktop terminals were located on the nursing station counter top.

Table 2.6. Hospital F Implementation Chronology

Date	Occurrence
April 1988	Signed contract
July 1988	CCU/ICU went live with med administration
March 1989	Converted to L.A.N. configuration
May 1989	Rehab, 7E and 7W Medical went live with VS, fluid balance, and med administration
July 1989	8E, 8W surgical went live with similar functions
August 1989	3E Detox, CDTS, and Oncology live
September 1989	5E Pediatrics and 5W Ortho live

The hospital utilizes the Baxter-Delta ADT, patient accounting, order entry, radiology, and respiratory systems. The ADT system is interfaced to CliniCom. The laboratory utilizes the Cerner system and pharmacy the Pharmakon system which is interfaced to Clini-Com. There are plans to interface to the laboratory system in the future. Nurses use the system and find it easy to use. They say it has moderate value. Physicians do not utilize the system at all. Nurse associates and clinicians use the system minimally and find it useful at times.

CONCLUSIONS

These six case studies represent approximately 10 percent of all installations nation-wide. The conclusion that can be drawn from these hospitals' experiences are as follows:

1. The decision time frames for these systems were fairly long. Many of the hospitals decided to trial test the approach on a pilot unit prior to signing an agreement with the vendor of choice. The length of the decision process reflects the cost of these systems, the limited number of installs that are fully operational, the newness of the companies in the market, and the hospital-wide philosophical changes which must occur. In other words, these systems are a major capital investment for an approach that is not commonly in use, offered by unestablished companies to healthcare professionals who must make adjustments to their way of thinking in order to use this approach to deliver care. No wonder there are so few sales given the number of years these systems have been on the market. The risks are high, thus a long evaluation period.

2. The implementation timeframes extend over multiple years. This is not uncommon for installation of major hospital-wide HIS systems. However, it seems with the bedside concept and certain types of functionality it offers, the learning curve is very long. Most of these systems are brought up piece-meal, nursing unit by nursing unit and function by function. This also adds to what appears to be a never ending implementation process. In addition, some of the case study hospitals were early pioneers who bought the original release of the

software. By the time they complete the installation of the initial release, they are ready to upgrade to the new release. This adds to the feeling of the never ending install.

3. The systems which have been implemented have a long way to go to be perceived as part of a fully integrated system. Many of these systems are not designed that way, but for greater acceptance in the future, this may be a must. Many of the hospitals are not even utilizing the full functionality offered by the vendor. Most have plans, but many have already run out of funds.

4. For the most part, users feel that the tangible and intangible benefits outweigh the costs of the technology. It can be stated from experience that the achievement of benefits must be managed, they do not just happen.

5. Physicians are not active users of these systems. They are principally utilized by nurses. When information is easy to retrieve in a format which is easy to interpret, physicians will interact with the terminals. Inputting into the system is an even more difficult goal. In any event, if the system slows down the physician as he/she makes rounds, they will not be interested in using it.

6. There is not one best place to install the terminal. From these case studies, the term "bedside computer systems" should be changed to "somewhere in the patient's room" computer systems.

3

Tackling the Technology

Robert Cort and Albert G. Crawford

To design and implement a point-of-care-based HIS, both clinical and systems managers must successfully address numerous issues. Certainly not the least of these issues are the technological requirements posed by such systems. This chapter focuses on such technical demands, ranging from network architecture to security file management.

In this chapter, we rely upon several basic observations and projections concerning the state-of-the-art of bedside-based HIS design, and the implications of such designs for hardware and other technical requirements:

1. HISs, like computer systems in general, have performance limitations, from hardware, software, or both.

2. The significance of the limitations inherent in a particular HIS depends on the functions which that HIS is designed to perform.

3. HISs are evolving to allow clinical personnel to access an electronic, and integrated, medical record, and to do so at the point of care, i.e., the bedside.

4. As HISs continue to develop in these directions, hospital managers and staff concerned with HIS design and implementation must address a number of technical and policy issues that arise, inevitably,

from the technology of the HISs and the requirements of the clinical personnel who will use them. Specifically, the operational requirements include:

- Fast response
- Convenient access, not only at the bedside and other points of care but also in remote locations such as offices and homes
- Constant or nearly constant system availability
- An optimal balance of access and security, so that authorized users are never disallowed access, and unauthorized persons are never allowed access
- Archival of records, to guarantee security and to allow relatively fast retrospective access to historical records for patient care, education, and research

This chapter reviews the state-of-the-art and emerging technologies that can be used to meet these requirements.

TYPOLOGY OF HOSPITAL INFORMATION SYSTEMS

HIS can be classified in a variety of ways: according to their hardware platform, database design, terminal location, type of user interface, degree of automation of documentation, and so forth. Rowland and Rowland (1985) write that seven design issues must be confronted in building an HIS:

1. Should the system(s) be departmental, serving departments individually, or should there be one comprehensive system interconnecting all departments throughout the hospital?
2. Should the system only transport information from place to place, or should all information on each patient's care be immediately available for retrieval and ready reference?
3. Should clerks enter information into the system; or should it be used directly by doctors, nurses, laboratory technologists, admitting personnel, etc.?

4. Should the hospital develop its own information system, or should it select one that has already been developed and proven elsewhere?

5. Should the hospital own and operate its own computer center, or should it contract for computer services from an external, shared center?

6. What computer technology should be employed—large mainframe computers, minicomputers, or microcomputers?

7. Should all computer purchases be part of a larger scheme for integrating computer systems throughout the hospital?

Although these will be open questions for any hospital choosing an HIS, it is important to recognize that the state-of-the-art HIS design assumes certain answers, for example, preferences for integrated systems instead of departmental ones, and for an electronic medical record rather than just order entry and charge capture. Although the various design dimensions are analytically separable, in practice, actual systems available for purchase tend to represent clusters of design choices, so that there is actually a relatively small number of types of systems available.

Thus, we have developed a typology, with six types, which is only as complex as necessary, given that it is derived from the systems actually developed and in use.

Not surprisingly, this typology is quite similar to those developed by other analysts, such as Rowland and Rowland (1985) and Fedorowicz (1982).

Discrete Manual Systems

Discrete manual systems are conventional, or nonautomated, departmental systems. They entail neither automation nor integration, e.g., nursing and lab departments whose operations are totally manual.

Discrete Automated Systems

Discrete automated systems are stand-alone systems which address the needs of only one department. There is automation within the department but no integration or even interfacing between departments; for example, nursing and lab operations are each computerized, but there is no electronic communication between them.

LAN-Based Automated Systems

There are various types of HISs that cross departmental boundaries. The type based on a local area network (LAN) is relatively loosely connected, in that it allows users to access the data in many separate departmental systems, but does not necessarily include specific interfaces, let alone an integrated database. Such networks typically are slow at retrieving results from different departmental systems, and provide little standardization across the various screens with which the user must interact. Recent developments, however, may provide increased speed and standardized inquiry screens. These capabilities, coupled with standards like HL-7, may eventually lead to very powerful LAN-based systems.

Centralized Order Entry Systems

The most basic type of interdepartmental database integration is order transmission, which may be accompanied by result transmission. These systems were usually designed primarily as charge capture systems and often require extensive modification in order to function as real patient care systems. Following Fedorowicz (1982), we can distinguish two levels of such systems:

A Level 1 system that includes ADT subsystem and a data collection message switching subsystem. On-line terminals are in place throughout the hospital for order entry, communication of the orders, and for charge capture. Periodically, once or twice a day, the system must be cleared of captured charges. The only permanent data base for the duration of the patient stay is the demographic data maintained by the ADT system.

A Level 2 system includes all the capability of a level 1 HIS but in addition maintains some archival structure for maintaining the patient medical record of orders, results, progress notes, etc. It also maintains data bases for ancillaries. As such, it can generate medication schedules, nursing care plans, cumulative lab results, etc. It can also provide a wealth of information upon inquiry, such as all active orders, medication profiles, uncompleted lab tests, etc.

The level 2 systems delineated by Fedorowicz actually fall into the remaining two categories.

Integrated Systems with Independent Modules

Integrated systems with independent modules are systems with a moderate degree of integration from department to department; processing is "distributed" across the various departmental central processing units (CPUs), and integration is accomplished through interfaces. There is usually a centralized database of information which is accessed by the doctors and nurses. This database duplicates the data in the ancillary systems. Although data is available, integration of function across departments, for instance, pharmacy versus nursing medication administration, is difficult.

Totally Integrated Systems

Totally integrated systems are systems with a high degree of interdepartmental integration, and with centralization of processing in one or more CPUs. The database is totally integrated, which means that all data related to a patient are stored in one place, and there is no duplication. All of the ancillaries share the same database, and functions performed by many different practitioners can all be tied together. Medication orders, pharmacist dispensing, nurse documentation of medication administration, and quality assurance review are all done on the same system, from any terminal, and data can be easily reviewed. Totally integrated systems make it easy for practitioners such as nurses to document observations or to review results from different ancillaries, and for technicians such as phlebotomists to report findings to their ancillary from any terminal.

SYSTEM ARCHITECTURE

HIS power and integration requirements have implications for system architecture. Thus, when a system selection committee chooses an

HIS with a certain level of functionality, it is also choosing, explicitly or implicitly, a certain type of system architecture. A review of the characteristics of the most common HIS architectures may serve to make such selection decisions better informed.

As delineated by Rowland and Rowland (1985), there are three common types of HIS processing designs: the large monolithic system (usually called a "mainframe machine") with a single CPU, a network using a large- or medium-size host central processor with additional attached processors, and mini- and microcomputer-based networks.

The advantages of the first type, with a monolithic design and single CPU, include its accommodation of a consolidated database and its processing efficiency, given such a database. Nevertheless, the technology has developed so that distributed networks with multiple CPUs can also maintain a consolidated database. Moreover, the monolithic design has several disadvantages: higher cost than the other alternatives, especially when fault tolerance is required; and inflexibility with respect to the addition of modular, i.e., departmental, systems requiring some other type of hardware.

In a network using a large- or medium-size host CPU, that processor performs data collection, consolidation, and some communication functions, whereas departmental modules operate on a variety of other CPUs linked through the network. In practice, these other CPUs may or may not be from the same manufacturer as the central CPU, depending on the hardware preferences of the different software vendors. Interfaces are necessary for the disparate CPUs to work together. The advantages of this type of system architecture lie in the ability of each ancillary to purchase the module that best suits its needs. Also, existing departmental systems can usually be interfaced into the network, thereby protecting those investments. The key disadvantage is that system maintenance is more difficult, with many different hardware and software vendors blaming one another for system problems. Another problem is that most of these types of systems simply interface, rather than integrate, the departments, which means that accessing various departmental functions, other than result reporting, often requires use of terminals attached to the departmental processor. For example, phlebotomists on the patient floor must locate a lab terminal to enter their information into the lab system, rather than simply accessing lab functions through any terminal connected to the integrated system.

There are at least three varieties of mini- and microcomputer networks: a communicating star network, a distributed star, and a distributed network. A communicating star network is basically a smaller version of a network using a large- or medium-size host CPU, as described above. A distributed star is similar, except that its central CPU is dedicated to controlling the other CPUs; the other functions are performed by other CPUs under the control of the central CPU. Finally, in a distributed network there is no specialization among the CPUs; the software dynamically allocates transactions among the CPUs and thus levels the load. The big advantage of a distributed network is that if a CPU fails, the system can still function, but at a reduced level. This built-in redundancy and backup usually justifies the added software cost of such a network. Another advantage of mini- and microcomputer networks is that hardware can easily and inexpensively be added to the network as use of the system grows.

REQUIREMENTS OF TOTALLY INTEGRATED HOSPITAL INFORMATION SYSTEMS

Rowland and Rowland (1985) draw on work by Whall (1982) to delineate the constraints imposed by two key factors, computer processing power and degree of automated information sharing, on the design options available to hospitals. Specifically, as Rowland and Rowland (1985) cite Whall, system planners must recognize various needs in making a hardware acquisition decision. Although these authors were not addressing bedside terminal based HISs per se, their list of user requirements is relevant to such implementations:

1. The number and size of application programs to be run concurrently
2. Number of on-line terminals and response times required
3. On-line data storage requirements
4. Interconnections to other processors, peripherals, and data communications lines

5. Growth potential without conversion
6. System backup and redundancy

The discussion that follows specifically addresses user requirements, or expectations, which must be met, and the technologies available to fulfill those requirements.

Fast Response

The first observation, and complaint, that many users make about a computer system concerns its response time. To understand the factors that influence response time, it is helpful to understand certain data processing concepts. The speed with which a CPU responds to a user's request and displays a screen full of data on a monitor is a function of several variables: the processing speed of the CPU per se, the total number of user requests at that time (including both "foreground jobs" and "background jobs"), the amount of data to be processed by those requests, whether the requested functions are options in the currently loaded program, the size of the other programs that must be loaded to perform the functions, the total amount of main memory in the CPU, the number of disk accesses required by the user's request, the speed of the disk(s), and the speed of data communications between the host and the user's terminal or personal computer.

The most commonly accepted definition of response time is the interval between when the "enter" key is pressed and when the first requested data element is displayed on the screen. Most HISs display each part of the screen as its processing is completed, so that the first result requested may be displayed in much less time than a second, although it may take several seconds to display the entire screen. Moreover, if the user request involves a considerable amount of disk accessing or processing, the total response time interval may be much longer. For instance, if the required results must be drawn from many different files or tables in the database, then the response time will increase accordingly.

A mainframe or minicomputer typically executes hundreds of thousands or millions of instructions per second, meaning that a single instruction may only require some billionths of a second to be executed. However, a single user request may entail thousands of instructions and also multiple disk accesses. Each access to a disk drive may require some thousandths of a second, enough time for several thousand instructions to be executed. Additionally, CPUs are designed not to wait during a long disk access, but rather to execute other instructions in the meantime. Thus, many users' requests can be processed simultaneously, optimizing total processing power.

On the other hand, if too many users make requests at the same time, response time may slow to several seconds. Among the solutions to this problem are a faster CPU, more or faster disk drives, or a combination of CPU and disk drive enhancements.

Alternatively, the database can be designed so that related data are stored together, so that they can be read together. However, this approach may be problematic, insofar as there may be no ideal way to organize the data. For instance, lab test results may be requested not only by patient, but also by test, by lab instrument, by accession number, by specimen number, and so forth.

Another alternative is to store data in multiple groupings. However, although retrieval is accelerated by this approach, it uses significantly more storage space, and the time to process the initial storage is increased; thus, the net improvement may be suboptimal. The compromise that is usually used is to write the data in one table and then to set up "cross reference" files with pointers to the initial data table. To improve response time even further, only the primary data table is written when the user enters the information; another program immediately begins to operate in the background to create all of the cross-reference pointers while the user is free to proceed to other requests. Although this makes it faster for the user entering the data, this simultaneous processing in the foreground and in the background requires almost the same level of system resources in toto, so that overall system processing may still be delayed.

Additionally, this approach causes a delay, of up to several minutes, before data can be accessed through the cross-references. For most applications, such as those involving registration data or routine lab test result entry and review, this delay is not a problem. However, for other applications, such as a stat lab where results must be retrieved quickly in various groupings, such a delay could produce serious operational problems.

Once the CPU has processed the request, the resulting data must be transmitted back to be displayed on the user's terminal or personal computer (PC) monitor. If the device is connected directly to the CPU, the communication speed is typically 9,600 bits per second (bps). Since it takes 8 bits to display a character, and since 20–30% of the data transmitted is required simply to control the terminal display, the effective transmission speed is approximately 900 characters per second. A typical screen display contains close to 500 characters, so it takes more than half a second just to send the display to the screen. Transmission of a full screen of graphics may require several seconds. If the data communications involves telephone lines or certain other types of networks, the transmission speed may be much slower. Specifically, a modem is required if a telephone line is to be used for access to the CPU. Most modems used on PCs today operate at 1,200 or 2,400 bps, which are only one-eighth or one-fourth as fast as the standard 9,600. With equipment operating at the slower—1,200 and 2,400 bps—rates, a standard screen of data may require several seconds to display and a screen of graphics may take correspondingly longer. Faster speeds are usually not essential; however, if speed is critical, it can be attained with faster modems, but at a higher cost. Clearly, the cost can become prohibitive as the number of users requiring high speeds increases, all other things being equal.

Acceptable Response Times for Different Uses and Users

The need for speed is determined by various factors. Clearly, patient acuity is an important determinant: An application designed for care of trauma patients or ICU patients must run faster than one for inpatients on a M/S unit. Additionally, the general functions of the HIS, and not just the characteristics of the patients, have a bearing on response time requirements. For example, a batch based order entry/charge capture system used by clerical personnel does not require as rapid a response time as an on-line system used for documentation by clinical personnel.

A general conclusion which can be made is that bedside systems invariably require relatively fast response. Addressing the specific requirements of HISs that are designed for use by physicians, Rowland and Rowland (1985) argue that system designers must guarantee that physicians do not encounter delays, resulting from either data input in particular or from overall system procesisng in general. Regarding the latter problem, that of overall response time, Rowland and Rowland (1985) state the following:

> Experience has shown that the response time to change from one display to the next should not exceed 0.5 seconds and that the time to retrieve data from a patient's record, format it, and present it should not exceed 3.0 seconds. These response times are within the "thinking time" of most physicians; little conscious slowing of activity should occur. (p. 5)

One final note is that response times guaranteed by vendors may not be appropriate indicators on which to base a system evaluation or a selection decision. Instead, discussions with current users of systems are more informative; following such discussions, those charged with the responsibility for system selection can discuss the issue with vendors in a more realistic and productive manner.

Convenient Access: Terminal Installation Considerations

Ten years ago, to install a terminal a technician would run a cable from the main computer room to the terminal location, install a special connector in the wall where the cable emerged, and link the terminal to the connector with a cable. Such cabling was, and frequently still is, a fairly expensive and time-consuming endeavor. Today, however, there are several alternative approaches to terminal installation, namely, data over voice (DOV) technology and LANs.

Data Over Voice Technology

DOV technology capitalizes on the fact that in almost any location where a terminal might be desired, there is already a telephone installed nearby. In DOV technology, the data signal is added to the analog voice signal on the twisted pair of telephone lines in such a way that it does not interfere with the conversation. At each user's workstation, a small device called a "multiplexor" is plugged into the telephone outlet, and both the telephone and the workstation are connected to that shared device and, thus, that telephone line. The multiplexors either combine the signals or separate them, as needed.

Transmission speeds in most DOV systems are limited to 9,600 or 19,200 bps; such speeds are usually adequate for terminals, but they may be too slow for some PC applications. It should be noted, however, that this technology will not work with the newer, all digital telephone systems.

Combining DOV technology with a data switch, which is similar to a telephone switch or PBX, creates a system that can be used to access multiple systems from a single terminal. It can also be used to provide load balancing for multiple CPUs, or even to connect PCs together. In many ways, this type of network looks and acts like a star LAN, the main difference being that a LAN usually operates at higher speeds, but gets bogged down if a large volume of data is transmitted between two devices.

Local Area Networks

A LAN typically has one of three configurations: a single long cable, or backbone; a ring of cable; or a star, which is a "hub" with many cables radiating out from it. All three configurations have various connectors located along the cable to allow attachment of computers, terminals, printers, and other devices. All LANs have the capability to transmit information at high speeds, including both data to display on a terminal and data files to transfer between computers. They can accommodate many terminals and/or PCs, and can allow these various workstations to share printers, modems, and other peripheral devices. To add a terminal to an older LAN, one had to take the LAN out of service for a short time while a new connector was added; however, recent developments have made this downtime unnecessary. LANs usually work very well for communications between PCs and printers or other peripheral devices, but large volumes of interactive terminal use can cause serious response time problems.

Over the last several years the power of high-speed LANs has become available over twisted-pair telephone lines. Most recent institutional telephone installations include three or four pair of wires at each jack, with only one or two pairs required for telephone service. One of the extra pairs can be used for high-speed LAN connections. The most common LAN installations using twisted pair wiring are star networks, which best take advantage of the existing telephone wiring. In these networks there is a "hub" which controls the LAN, located in or near the telephone room; and all of the data lines radiate out from this controller in a "star" arrangement, using the telephone lines. The benefits of such an implementation include both ease of initial installation and ease of expansion. However, for a large install-ation, a powerful central unit is required. This is costly; and if the unit fails, all communication is lost.

The central processing units and terminals sold by some HIS vendors may only operate on certain types of network hardware or software, may only operate on certain media, e.g., coaxial cable, or may be subject to other restrictions. Such constraints on the options available to a hospital can lead to sub-optimal HIS choices.

Additionally, any system which allows point-of-care documenta-tion, or an electronic medical record, will require a relatively high number of terminals, compared with a system with more limitations on the logistics or level of documentation. An HIS should be selected to guarantee that both initial installation, and subsequent expansion or relocation of workstations, will be fast and easy.

System Availability

There are no perfect HISs; sooner or later, every system, including manual as well as automated ones, will suffer a failure of some sort, and operations will come to a halt. Since computer systems are often powerful and can support many different types of operations simul-taneously, a system "crash" can affect a multitude of people. The ramifications of a system outage depend on the extent of computeriza-tion, the length of the outage, and the appropriateness of the disaster recovery procedures, manual or automated, which can be employed. If the system performs critical functions, the hardware should be configured to minimize the likelihood of failure in the first place or to minimize its impact, i.e., its duration. Systems of this type are called "fail-safe" or "high-availability" systems.

Fail-safe systems are designed with a high degree of redundancy, so that the system as a whole will not fail even if a component fails. Storage media, communication controllers, and processing compo-nents are, to a greater or lesser degree, duplicated. If a device fails, its duplicate takes over the function. Some of these systems are so "fault-tolerant" that users may be unaware of the substitution.

In contrast, high-availability systems contain hardware and operating system features that expedite system recovery after a failure. Instead of duplicating all of the key hardware components, which is very expensive, high-availability systems are designed so that they can easily recover from a failure and can be restored to operation in a matter of minutes or, at most, hours.

Perfect fault-tolerance is an ideal to which computer system designers aspire; however, the cost associated with such perfection is difficult to justify in cost benefit terms.

System Availability Requirements of Bedside Terminal Systems

If the ultimate goal of a patient-care computer system is complete automation of the medical record, the hardware requirements are quite different from those of a system that merely automates one or several functions, for example, order entry or financial processing. In earlier generations of patient-care system implementations, only order entry, and perhaps result reporting, were automated. The rationale for developing such systems was to facilitate a cost-based reimbursement system and, specifically, to allow for charge capture. In such systems, any order or item that has a charge associated with it is entered into the system, and then a batch of such charges is transmitted to the financial computer system. In some cases, patient transfers and other patient data are recorded in the system, but usually only to support financial functions.

Order entry is generally performed in batch mode; that is, nurses or clerks transcribe batches of orders from order forms completed by physicians. The computer system verifies the orders, transmits charge records to the financial system for billing purposes, and prints a copy of the order form in the appropriate ancillary department. The hardware required for such batch processing is minimal: one or several terminals at each nursing station, a printer and maybe a terminal in each ancillary department, and a host computer designed for the level of batch processing generated by such a configuration of input and output devices.

When a simple order entry system of this type goes down, it creates relatively few problems in all but the largest hospitals. In the event of a system failure, orders are carried by hand from the nursing stations to the ancillaries, and charge entry is postponed until the system is restored to operation. Although such adaptations are annoying in small institutions and somewhat daunting in large ones, there is little risk of serious clinical or financial repercussion. For example, stat orders are still processed quickly, and results are still reported on paper.

Such order entry systems have seldom included high-availability or fail-safe features. Typically, in fact, they are taken down for a few hours each night while operators back-up disks and a disk crash may result in 12–24 hours of downtime, a period of unavailability that is generally deemed acceptable.

From the standpoint of reliability requirements, stand-alone departmental systems generally fall into the same category as simple order entry systems; that is, they have neither high-availability nor fail-safe systems. Enough paper is routinely printed during result processing so that if and when the system fails, the technicians can continue processing manually. Results are typically printed as soon as they become available, and the only data that might be lost are results of tests completed just before the crash. If the system provides for result reporting at nursing stations or other convenient locations on the patient floors, physicians and nurses will have to cope with the inconvenience of telephoning ancillaries for results. Of course, in a high-volume application, the burden of such phone calls on an ancillary might compromise its ability to provide test results in a timely fashion, particularly if the outage were severe. As a result, large ancillary departments may consider installing optional hardware to support high-availability, or even fail-safe operation.

If a patient care system typically provides results on-line, with printed copies distributed at most once a day, then system downtime can have a severely adverse impact on patient care. If the medical record is totally electronic, with no parallel paper chart at all, losing access to the system for even a few hours can impair patient care. If scheduling functions are also performed on-line, additional aspects of patient care will also be handicapped.

Therefore, an electronic medical record system must be designed so that it will never go down for routine functions like daily system backups, and the hardware must be as fail-safe as possible. It should be possible to perform system backups, routine diagnostics, trouble shooting, and even CPU and disk upgrades without taking down the system. Although many vendors claim that their systems operate on multiple processors or on processors with "good track records," system managers should be careful. They should obtain from vendors a complete description of what system features become unavailable when one of the processors or disks fails, and what corrective actions may be taken in the event of all imaginable failure scenarios.

Disaster Recovery

Disasters may arise from both human and nonhuman sources. Neutralization of human threats is the topic of the section on security. A full treatment of control of the physical environment is beyond the scope of this chapter; nevertheless, a few words are in order on disaster planning for bedside-based HISs.

Because the integrated on-line medical record is such an important part of patient care, a fire, flood, or other disaster in the computer room, resulting in loss of the system for several days, can be a disaster on the patient floor. Realistically, the only protection against this sort of failure is some kind of remote processing capability. Remote processing can be done in one of two ways:

- Restoring operations as quickly as possible in an off-site backup facility, either one designated by the HIS hardware or software vendor or one designed for that purpose by a third-party firm can be accomplished. Hospitals using "shared systems" may have no need for disaster recovery of the type described here; nevertheless, it should also be mentioned that most of the high-functionality options assumed herein, i.e., point-of-care system access, and an integrated electronic medical record, are seldom supported as part of shared systems.

- Restoring operations as quickly as possible through hardware and/or software maintained in a separate location at the hospital site itself can be accomplished.

Regardless of what specific hardware-oriented disaster recovery approach is selected, a software-oriented recovery approach is necessary as well. The most important recommendation that can be made here is to develop, implement, and scrupulously conduct appropriate software backup procedures, including off-site storage.

ARCHIVING OF MEDICAL RECORDS

One advantage of on-line patient records is the capability for rapid retrieval of data from previous hospital admissions and clinic visits. A complete historical medical record, for tens or hundreds of thousands of patients, however, requires a large amount of storage space. Traditionally, large volumes of data that were not accessed constantly were archived on magnetic tape. Tape is very inexpensive, and large amounts of data can be stored on a single reel, but retrieving the data from tape can be very time-consuming. There is no way to simply read the piece of data that you want from the middle of the tape. Instead, the entire tape must be read until the piece of data you are looking for is found. If the data in question is at the end of the tape, this can take up to several minutes. This is in addition to the time spent finding the correct tape, which must be located in a large library of such tapes, and the time spent loading the tape onto a tape drive, so that its contents can be accessed by the machine. Aside from the cost of the labor involved, there is an additional problem in using tape for an on-line medical records system: Typical time delays of 5–10 minutes before data can be retrieved are probably unacceptable. There are two technologies that may provide an alternative to magnetic tape: high-density magnetic disks and optical disks.

High-Density Magnetic Disks

Magnetic disks are the direct access storage devices (DASDs) used by most computers today. A simple version of the magnetic disk is the floppy disk used with most personal computers; a more advanced version is the hard disk located inside many PCs. Magnetic disks are flat, circular, magnetized devices, which look much like a phonograph record. The disks are spun at a high speed, and a sensitive magnetic head reads or writes the data. On large computers, the disks are very similar to those found in PCs, except that the data density and rotation speed are greater. Where a PC floppy disk stores approximately one million characters, or bytes, of data 1 MB, a large computer disk system may store in excess of 20 billion bytes of data (20 gigabytes or GB). High-density magnetic disks have been available for many years, but the cost per megabyte of storage has been very high compared to tape storage. The pressure from the mass marketing of the personal computer has recently brought the cost per megabyte of magnetic disk storage down to a point where disk storage of large volumes of data is becoming quite attractive, even though it is certainly not as inexpensive as tape storage.

Optical Disks

Optical disks look very much like the compact discs (CDs) available for audio systems. The difference is that an optical disk used for a computer can store much larger quantities of data, and can be written on. A disadvantage for most potential uses of optical disks, however, is that they are "WORM" disks (Write Once, Read Many), which can only be written on once. Recent advances have produced optical disks that can be erased and rewritten many times. Still, for the archival purposes of on-line medical records, a WORM disk will be satisfactory. In fact, a medium that allows information to be written only once and then not erased has an advantage from the perspectives of data security and risk management.

Optical disks have been available for several years, and it has been assumed, given that they use light and lasers for writing and reading, that the density would be much greater, and the ultimate cost per megabyte would be significantly lower than those of magnetic disks. As mentioned above, however, there have recently been great strides in reducing the cost per megabyte of magnetic disk storage. At this time, it is not clear which technology will eventually prove most cost effective for archiving data on-line.

SECURITY

Issues

One of the greatest benefits of a bedside-based HIS, particularly one with an electronic medical record, is the convenience, speed, and depth of access to the patient chart. Results may be instantly and automatically displayed, trended, graphed, and analyzed, and orders entered, by various clinicians, at the patients bedside, as well as at a myriad of other locations, both on the hospital grounds and beyond. However, where bedside terminals are the means of access to the patient chart, especially where it is an electronic chart, there are profound implications for the quality of patient care, on the one hand, and for patients' privacy, on the other hand. Thus, accessibility brings along with it a corresponding burden of security. There must be mechanisms to restrict access so that only those individuals authorized to look at certain portions of the chart can examine them and, even more importantly, to prevent unauthorized order entry into the chart.

Hospitals are distinctive, if not unique, in the speed, or immediacy, with which users must be able to gain access to the computer system and its data review and order entry capabilities. It is hard to argue that matters are ever more critical than they are in medical emergencies. Because immediate access to data is often essential, and because care must be provided on a 24-hour-a-day basis, data must be accessible by, and ordering capability available to, a wide range of unspecified clinical personnel. Heightening the dilemma of access to, versus protection of, private information is the extraordinary cost of not allowing access to patient information immediately on demand. Unlike financial transactions, the risks and potential costs involved in not providing access can be greater than those involved in providing inappropriate access. For example, if a patient were in a clinical crisis and the computer system were to allow that patient's medical record to be seen only by a specific list of medical practitioners, who happened to be unavailable, the patient might receive inadequate or inappropriate emergency care.

When an HIS is implemented, decisions must be made regarding a number of access issues: most importantly, who will be allowed to use the system, and what information, and what other rights, e.g., order entry, will be available to them. There are also more specific issues such as whether to permit off-site chart review by physicians, and off-site order entry and, if such functions are allowed, how to manage such remote access.

Solutions

Security for all types of access to the system should be controlled through the database, i.e., through a security file describing the electronic medical record access rights of hospital employees and admitting physicians. This mechanism, in turn, should be governed by hospital policies. Most modern HISs control access through user codes and passwords, and some require a physical device like a card or a key. A system using cards works the same way that an automated teller machine works. The user is required to insert the card into a reader connected to the terminal, and then to enter a password to access the system. The user must have both the card and knowledge of the password to gain access. This eliminates the possibility of someone observing an authorized user entering his code and then signing on as that user. More elaborate schemes involving automatic identification through fingerprint and retina pattern matching are also available, and they provide tighter security, particularly because there is no card that can be lost or stolen; however, such elaborate systems are also much more costly.

The level of system security can be controlled not only by access method, as discussed above, but also by terminal location and time of day. For example, an HIS should allow for restricting access via terminals in a given department to the normal working hours of that department.

In most systems the weak link in the security chain is the access allowed to users who wish to use the system from a remote location by using a modem. "Hackers," those who seek to gain access for amusement or revenge, can cause major problems and are a substantial threat to system security. However, even on relatively unprotected systems, it is not as easy to gain entry as some writers would have us believe. Relatively simple hardware- and software-based solutions exist to guard against even the most persistent hacker. Frequently, the hacker is a disgruntled exemployee, and simply deleting security codes of former employees in a timely manner prevents many problems.

The surest method of preventing connections by unauthorized users is to disallow any access from remote locations. A more moderate approach, requiring all remote users to use leased lines, addresses the problem, but this may be too expensive a solution for general application. A leased line is essentially a telephone line that allows only one connection, from one user to the host computer. There is no way to gain access in such a system unless one is physically at the device using that leased line. If there are many users scattered throughout many remote locations, however, this option becomes very expensive.

If general dial-up capability is the only practical approach for remote access, then precautions must be taken. One of the most popular precautionary techniques is automatic call-back. This solution identifies the caller, looks up the caller's telephone number in an internal table, and then calls that number back, to ensure that the caller is in fact who he or she claims to be. Because it is the HIS that creates the working telephone line connection, access will only be granted to numbers predefined within the HIS. This approach has been used successfully for a number of years; however, its viability is decreasing as a result of new features available on private telephones. One such option, available to most consumers, is call-forwarding, which can be activated remotely. A hacker could make a call to an authorized user's phone, forward that phone to his own, and then make a call to the HIS and attempt to sign on as the authorized user. When the HIS calls back the authorized user's phone to establish the connection, the call is forwarded to the hacker's phone. One solution to this problem is not allowing access from phones with the call-forwarding option.

Other methods of preventing unauthorized system access over telephone lines include encrypting the data signals, installing hardware that sends special signals on the line, and other, more exotic solutions. For integrated patient care systems, most of these approaches may be "overkill." In any event, the deciding factors in choosing security technologies will probably be hospital policies and governmental and Joint Commission on the Accreditation of Healthcare Organizations (JCAHO) regulations.

SUMMARY AND CONCLUSIONS

All HISs have limitations. The significance of the limitations of a particular HIS depends on its functions. The guiding premises of this chapter have been that, in state-of-the-art HISs, clinical personnel can access an electronic medical record, and can do so at the point of care, i.e., the bedside, and that as HISs continue to develop in this direction, those concerned with their design and implementation must be careful to confront the technical and policy issues that arise inevitably from their technology and from the requirements of their users, especially clinical personnel.

Specifically, users' operational requirements include the following:

- Fast response
- Convenient access, at the bedside, at other points of care, and in offices and homes
- Constant or nearly constant system availability
- An optimal balance of access and security, so that authorized users are never denied access, while unauthorized persons are never allowed access
- Archival of records, to guarantee security and to allow fast access to historical records

Various state-of-the-art and emerging technologies and approaches can be used to address these issues:

- HIS selection to guarantee appropriate system architecture and database design
- Implementation of enhancements to CPUs and storage media to optimize performance, i.e., response time
- Use of LAN and/or DOV technology to maximize the cost effectiveness of data communications
- Employment of "fail-safe" and "high-availability" HIS components to prevent downtime, or to reduce it to an absolute minimum
- Institution of conscientious backup procedures for both programs and data
- Careful planning of disaster recovery procedures
- Development of security policies and techniques, including use of multiple levels of security along every path of access to the HIS

Careful attention to these issues, and use of appropriate techniques for addressing them, can prevent a host of problems and make the implementation, and continued operation, of a sophisticated HIS a much smoother process.

REFERENCES

Fedorowicz, J. (1982) Hospital information systems: are we ready for case mix applications? *Health Care Management Review VIII*, 4.

Hafner, K. M., et al. (1988) Is your computer secure?: hackers, viruses, and other threats, *Business Week*, Aug. 1, 64–70.

Hammond, W. E., and W. W. Stead. (1988) Bedside terminals: an overview (Editorial), *MD Computing*, V 1, 5–6.

Rowland, H. S., and B. L. Rowland. (1985) *Hospital Software Sourcebook*. Rockville, MD: Aspen Publishers.

Whall, D. E. (1982) Choosing an information system that fits both the hospital's needs and its capabilities. In B. I. Blum (Ed.) 5, *Proceedings of the Sixth Annual Symposium on Computer Applications in Medical Care,* 406–408. IEEE Computer Society Press, Washington, D.C.

4

Practical Considerations

Patricia McNeal

This chapter deals with many of the practical considerations surrounding bedside computer technology. Making the decision to purchase a bedside system is an infinitely more complex problem than making decisions to purchase any other type of hospital information system. The reasons for this are as complicated as understanding your particular institution's documentation and communications chains and as simple as envisioning spilled apple juice.

SPACE

Space is indeed "the final frontier" in most hospitals. Space is carefully planned, mapped out, and used to the last available inch, jealously guarded, rarely available just for the asking, and never where you need it. Space can be a critical consideration for those contemplating bedside terminal purchase. Where are you going to put it?

Where Will It Fit?

After deciding which of the available systems best meets your institution's clinical needs, the size and shape of the terminals become an issue. The measurements and configurations of the various data input centers will assist you in determining location possibilities within the confines of the average patient room. And what works in one room, won't necessarily work in all of them because of the vagaries of construction and usage.

Those planning bedside installations as part of an overall renovation or building project have the most attractive and utilitarian option available to them, making the system part of an in-wall construction process. Cabinetry can be designed to allow air flow, maintenance access, and the optimal wall-flush mounting of the terminal screen face.

The top of the standard bedside cabinet is rarely an option because of all of the other "traditional" functions it performs (e.g., holder of juice, tissues, water pitcher, dressing supplies and irrigation trays, etc.). Space between beds may be an option for placing a dedicated computer table, but watch where bedside curtains fall in terms of assuring both user access and patient privacy. Consider too that the table should only be large enough to hold the computer and keyboard, if any. Vacant, flat surfaces in patient rooms are immediate targets for an incredible amount and variety of things, most of which will be hazardous to the life and well-being of the computer. Additionally, they are a catcher of dust that will require cleaning.

Dependent upon room design and layout, partially remote locations may be your best option. For instance, rooms designed with vestibules can be equipped with cabinetry or mechanisms to hold the terminal, thereby providing in-room access. Existing eye-level storage may provide the ideal location if it can be properly converted to the needs of the terminal without loss of critical supply storage space. Keep in mind that stretcher, wheelchair, and emergency equipment access demands are always your primary consideration in location determinations. The health-care team must always be able to maneuver necessary patient care technology within the room confines, without undue delay or constraints.

Contemplation of room size and limits often lead to the thought that it would be nice to be able to pull the terminal down from somewhere overhead during use and then push it up and away afterwards—using skyhooks, as it were. As of this writing, a single company on the west coast is prototyping this sort of mechanism for business use. Because it is prototypical rather than mass-produced, however, the cost per room makes large-scale implementation financially impractical. Time and more widespread experience with bedside computerization may rectify this problem, however, since the "skyhook" image remains a popular one in most people's minds.

Commercially available swing-arm mechanisms can allow placement options that move the terminal from side to side while providing limited up and down movement as well. Some institutions have used this type of arm to optimize space by placing the terminals at eye level in the arm down or pulled out position and out of the way when in the up or pushed back position. Swing-arms also provide the option of swiveling the terminal display face to either bedside for patient education usage. A cautionary note is injected, however: Placement using swing-arms must keep heights and positioning in mind at all times to prevent inadvertent user injury. Also keep in mind that custom alterations may be necessary to hold the keyboard and cabling, dependent upon the mechanism and system chosen. As always, remember that all of this must be kept clean, dry, and dust-free on an ongoing basis. Terminals should never be placed over radiators or sinks where excessive heat or water splash can lead to otherwise unnecessary repair costs and related access delays.

A basic shelving arrangement can be the most utilitarian and cost-effective approach to terminal placement in your particular situation. Considerations when installing shelving include the strength of the materials used and the type of support structure installed with reference to the weight and size of the terminal. Placing the shelving at eye level for the average standing user is one approach but can lead to the terminal being too high for some and too low for others; placement at eye level for the seated user imposes the need for seating as well as the shelving.

Interaction Approaches

There are additional decisions to be made when selecting your system in terms of keyboard, light-pen or hand-held data entry methods. There are pluses and minuses to all three system types.

Hand-held data entry systems are portable, and the majority of available systems are lightweight and convenient for the most part. On the downside are problems like the ease of mishandling the small, readily concealed entry mechanism. Going through trash or soiled linen searching for an inadvertently misplaced hand-held tool can be messy and annoying at best, time-consuming and unproductive at worst. Theft/loss could become a common occurrence if hand-held tools are left unprotected in unsecured areas, since anyone could rightly or wrongly assume they contain usable/salable parts worth misappropriating.

Light-pens are a user-friendly option but can be an expensive system component when viewed from a loss and breakage standpoint. Since they are small and need to be stored somehow at the terminal site, user care and handling become pivotal decision-making parameters. Placement, cords, and holders must account for the potential for pens being dropped into nearby sinks, trash, or simply against cabinets or the floor. Pens that can be unplugged at the terminal site might become pocket property if the users run across too many terminals where pens are unavailable or not working properly.

Keyboards usually offer the widest range of data entry capabilities. But unless your system is heavily menu-driven, all of your users must be at least minimally keyboard literate or tolerant of the "hunt and peck" syndrome. Keyboards are probably the least damage-prone of the three options, but plastic key covers and velcro fasteners are good investments to prevent unnecessary dust and debris buildup, spills, and damage from being dropped. Sticky apple juice knocked across a keyboard can be an irreparable occurrence.

Substance Problems

Keep in mind that true bedside placement has implications beyond user access, and finding the right mechanisms and sufficient space. The number and variety of various substances to be found at the average patient bedside is impressive. Patients eat, drink, and take care of an alarming number of bodily functions in that small confined space. "Normal" spills like juice and cracker crumbs pale against the significance of fluids like Dakins' solutions (diluted chlorine bleach); tincture of benzoin (an incredibly sticky, thick brown fluid still occasionally in use as a skin protectant); and tube feeding solutions (high glucose content, thick and nearly impossible to clean up). Body secretions and excretions often fly and splatter; and the various containers, dressings, and coverings get laid down in odd and inappropriate locations at times. This brings up the issue of keeping the terminal sufficiently clean to pass infection control muster. True bedside placement creates a whole new set of problems in terms of handling isolation patients. You can't guarantee that a practitioner won't handle the patient then the terminal without pausing to wash their hands; and the cleansing process between patients may be less than thorough. Slightly remote locations (i.e., across from the foot of the bed; in the alcove next to the bathroom; in the vestibule to the room) and protective keyboard and/or even terminal covers, etc. are superior approaches to the problems of protecting the equipment from inadvertent contaminated handling and excessive food, fluid, and abuse exposure.

COMMUNICATIONS AND SYSTEMS ISSUES

Understanding the institution's "culture" and "climate" as outlined in the previous chapter will go far in assisting you with the issue of determining who needs what, how, where, and when. The problem, of course, is that now you literally can have it all. Every piece of data entered on the patient chart is now available for collation, sifting, measurement, and recording in some report somewhere. Deciding what you want and who should have access to this massive collection of data is as large a decision as making the one to purchase the system in the first place.

Structuring Data Retrieval

Initially, as you go through the various systems, you should keep a basic roster of information in your head (preferably also on paper) with regard to current reporting relationships, data needs, and requirements. What do you already have that is irreplaceable/ unchangeable/"can't-do-business-without-it"? Alternatively, what have you always wanted that you haven't been able to get your hands on due to the need to hand collate and abstract the information? Both lines of inquiry are pivotal decision-making parameters.

Not all systems will be able to give you exactly the report format you're accustomed to. Keep this in mind when reviewing the available report writer functions. How flexible is the master menu selection tree? If you're locked into strictly the reports the system automatically provides, are they adequate to your needs? Do they give you all the information you want in a format that your usual audience will be able to comprehend and use? The need to adhere to certain reporting guidelines because of familiarity is a dependence you may have to get over when facing the magnitude of system overhaul. Remember, however, that most of these systems will free up a tremendous amount of time currently spent manually collating such numbers, facts, and figures. You may be able to reallocate this time to a productive restructuring of the computer-generated information to your current format if you decide that is necessary to your particular climate and culture. Some systems however do provide sufficient flexibility and report writing capabilities to meet even the most demanding user's needs and wish list.

Attempt to prioritize your reporting needs according to "Must Have," "Would be nice to have," and "Wouldn't it be great if" classifications. This sorting will cull out the currently existing reports that can be condensed or done away with due to obsolescence. You may be surprised to discover the volume and types of reports being generated throughout your institution. It is always something of a revelation just how duplication of effort and data goes on in even the smallest institutions. It's rare that such information is deliberately hoarded, but frequently an exigency creates a report that somehow continues to propagate and regenerate until it's an accepted part of the environment. Once a report is available, it's often difficult to do away with it. The changeover to an HIS report generation format affords the institution an excellent opportunity for needs assessment and dissolution of some of the paper dragons that haunt the corridors of so many hospitals.

The new spector awaiting those installing HIS is that suddenly you can literally have just about any report you ever dreamed of. This "Info-Glut" is a common business phenomenon that few clinical people have been exposed to. Hospital personnel are generally not accustomed to having immediate access to statistics, rates, raw numbers, and rapidly calculated occurrence reports. Since the business-at-hand is that of caring for patients, paperwork and documentation are almost always sadly last on the priority lists. However, many aspects of paperwork are as important as direct patient care, in that information concerning the patient must be properly communicated. Because of that, and in some cases in spite of it, the medical record as the sole source of information has often stymied institutional efforts to gain access to necessary report data. Even with that problem, hospitals produce alarming amounts of statistics and reports that are gathered through a painstaking manual reading and abstraction process that uses many hours of time and energy. Given that such emphasis is placed on the process in a manual environment, it does not take great imagination to envision what could happen when suddenly you can get any combination of items you'd like simply by structuring the report and making the appropriate request. Information overload can be the devastating result of lack of planning and foresight in this area.

Structuring the entire data retrieval process right from the start is the single best method of combating incipient info glut. Awareness and utilization of standard terminology, as well as requiring certain fields of information like acknowledgments, sign-offs, and particular data pieces will keep the overall process streamlined and controlled. It is also the simplest and surest way to assure that desired data is available for the end point user. Keying into the types of reports required in your institution and making your report specifications clear from the beginning of the implementation is probably the only way to keep panic from setting in when the data output process finally begins.

Access Issues

Beyond determining what data should be collected comes the decision concerning who should have access, when, and how. The entire security question relative to computer systems is raised to exponentially increased importance in the case of terminals providing access to confidential patient and institutional information at the bedside. You have suddenly placed all of your institution's files in unmonitored locations that do not lend themselves to supervision by any level of personnel. Bedside terminals also means access in physician lounges for data retrieval and review. It can also mean terminals anywhere you decide they're a necessity. The ramifications of this become house-staff on-call areas: Do you allow remote order entry and risk the M.D. not physically visiting the patient? Or is the speed and convenience of providing easier access more desirable? And is placement in a totally unmonitorable area going to increase your hardware loss costs? There are ways to answer all of these issues given sufficient consideration and thought. Physician access might be best monitored by way of allowing only data review access, *not* order entry from remote locations. And lock systems can be placed to minimize the risk of hardware loss.

The larger question in all of this becomes the risk of data confidentiality loss through carelessness, piracy, and plain nosiness. Terminals left in a data receipt mode without proper sign-off can be accessed by unauthorized personnel. Automatic defaults within certain time constraints of nonuse will be of major assistance in these cases. "Nosiness" is best defeated through well-defined security clearances that define access paths throughout the system and block unauthorized usage. Some users have reported employee review of files on other employees who have been patients to get birth dates and addresses.

Piracy is an area that has not been well addressed in HIS implementations thus far, but about which speculation is clearly possible. Where now one has to cull through piles and piles of paper to obtain such figures as infection and complication rates, consider the potential impact of merely accessing the system and asking for the data directly, and receiving it in mere seconds. How admissible such data would be in a court of law is clearly arguable, but, nonetheless, that information could give litigation-hungry clients unwelcome ammunition and the incentive to look further into records and data that *is* admissible. It becomes clear, then, just how important the installation and enforcement of a well-defined user security system is. Encoded badges with employee identification have been utilized with varying degrees of success dependent upon the institution's willingness to enforce rules against "trading" of badges, and loss-control policies. The second layer of protection is normally a numeric or password system designed to change with regularity despite the average human being's tendency to forget such items.

Security level decisions are the logical starting point. Analyze the options each system offers you—the more flexibility you have, the better your chances of protecting your database from inadvertent or even deliberate unauthorized access. Each different type of employee should have data access restricted by virtue of their job classification and its needs. Report writer functions should be strictly reserved for designated administrative personnel.

The second level of security access is more familiar to most people. Passwords and numbers have made their way into just about everyone's lives at some level whether through a bank card or a home PC.

Policies on use of passwords should clearly and distinctly prohibit "sharing" of passwords in order to promote the proper employee attitude and environment: one cognizant and respectful of the power of confidentiality and privacy matters.

DOCUMENTATION AND LEGALITIES

Documentation and legalities were briefly touched upon in the last section on access and security issues. They merit a fuller discussion simply because of several recurring issues in hospital documentation and because of some of the legality potentials raised by electronic database collection.

Defining Current Usage

How your current patient record is utilized will assist you in projecting how your electronic record will be used. Movement to a computerized data entry system will not, repeat will not, correct all of your current omissions and misusages. The issues that *will* disappear are the legibility, timing, and dating problems that plague all handwritten records. Quite simply, the computer is capable of dating and timing all entries for each user on a consistent basis and also of making the data output totally and completely legible. This does not correct the problems of late chart entries or poor grammar. Indeed, since the computer does a totally accurate timing and dating of each entry as it occurs new problems can arise. Many practitioners, particularly nurses, are accustomed to doing charting entries at the end of the shift rather than as events occur. This backtiming to reflect the real time at which the charted information was applicable is customary in many settings and often dictated by the demands upon the practitioner's time. As previously noted, paperwork is almost always a last priority for clinicians. Check to see whether your system allows for clinicians. Check to see whether your system allows the practitioner to enter a specific time the event occurred. And keep in mind that the fact that the capability exists does not assure that it will be used; you are once again faced with chart entries recorded at a time often significantly later than when they actually applied to the patient. It may be possible to make it a required entry in order to proceed through the rest of the documentation process. This is a system feature to note carefully in view of the potential legal ramifications. Consider for instance how experts currently piece together events surrounding a patient fall. All timed entries are laid out on a flow chart surrounding the time of the fall: vital signs, medications, I/O entries, progress notes, etc. These times are then used to demonstrate the presence or absence of health-care personnel monitoring of the patient at the time of the fall. Other factors are of course taken into the court's consideration, but if all of your documentation for a shift is typically written at the end of the shift now, it will automatically be *timed* as end of the shift by the computer if no steps are taken to override or clarify when the events reflected actually occurred.

The problem of unclear sentence structure and phrasing errors will not be cured by most systems. Indeed, some may compound the problems by forcing certain entries to be made according to a format the practitioner is not accustomed to using. Heavily menu-driven systems may alleviate some of these issues, but may restrict recording of unusual occurrences to strictly keystruck entries that require planning, forethought, and keyboard literacy as well. Most hospital quality assurance offices have a file of "funny" or unusual entries they have come across in the manually written charts—the illegible, the impossible, the anatomically curious. Many have found these files increasing in size when the additional complication of computers is added to the already complex process of recording and interpreting human thought and observation.

How your institution's current forms are used and structured must be compared to the availability and structure of the computer system's format. If certain forms are not well used now and do not reflect the type and quality of documentation you want from your record, do not perpetuate the problem by simply reproducing your current documentation system in the computer.

Alternatively, do not allow the computer system to overhaul parts of your documentation system that work well and already give you exactly what you need and want. All of this takes tremendous amounts of time and planning in terms of system assessment and user input. This cost factor is one usually underestimated by both the computer system seller and the buyer. Remember that every new "fix" you put into the system in terms of correcting an existing documentation problem may cost you end-user time to implement; if your clinicians do not currently have good charting habits and you choose to force correction through requiring certain items or forms, you will be adding time to the current charting process. The end result, of course, is that your records should be more accurate, but you have the other costs to consider in terms of user education and time consumed.

The progress note is probably the single most difficult item for computer systems to address appropriately and simply. Making huge menu-driven progress note sections requires a detailed analysis of current user patterns. Simply allowing direct keyboard entry to all progress notes can be daunting from the already mentioned perspectives of keyboard literacy and normal grammatical errors. Voice activation for direct transcription is still not technologically possible despite industry enthusiasm and user eagerness. Recording such entries verbally for later transcription, as is currently done in most places for things like operative and discharge notes, places an unfair burden on those trying to care for the patients at the bedside awaiting consults and information. Such delays could cause the caregivers to revert to a heavily verbal exchange system where they record things only when forced to. Computerization of progress notes will, in all likelihood, remain a difficult problem for all systems until direct transcription from voice activation is practical.

Access Issues

Tight control of user access should assist in negating the issue of "borrowed" security badges and passwords, but it will probably not cure all the potential problems. Dependent upon the type of system selected and where terminals are located, a myriad of possibilities arise. In current manual systems, there are already problems with co-signing of such items as medical student and physician assistant orders. Consider the system issues that arise when such order entry capability is electronic: It is infinitely easier to sign off on a terminal than to manually place a signature at the bottom of an order sheet. There is a simplicity to electronic signature that belies its impact; it simply does not have the same feel as placing one's signature on paper. Hence, it may result in cursory rather than critical reviews; it may be the ultimate rubber stamp.

Electronic signatures for medications are accepted in most states, but it does bear checking with your government offices to assure that your state does indeed give full faith and credit to electronic sign-off. Some states have specific filing requirements similar to the handling of physician signature stamps that must be complied with for the pharmacy to be able to accept the order as a valid physician prescription.

Order entry from areas removed from the patient's bedside creates another dimension of difficulty with assuring proper monitoring. Consider the problems created by orders generated by weary housestaff who do not make time to visit the bedside—terminals can be located in physician lounges, housestaff oncall quarters, or physician offices remote to the hospital. This can lead to orders based on phone conversation that may or may not contain accurate assessment data. Although it is not advisable or wise for a physician to base treatment on such information, the reality is that they do just that. But current manual systems generally enforce the physician presence at the patients' bedside within a set time period in order to write for verbally ordered treatments. Absent such a requirement, the in-person follow-up just may not occur. Such contingencies can be remedied by limiting remote terminals to emergency order entry and/or data review only. Some systems also offer the capability of recording where an order originated and requiring at-the-bedside cosignatures within certain time periods to assure in-person follow-up.

Patient Confidentiality

Confidentiality was noted briefly in a previous section. It is raised again here simply because its importance cannot be overemphasized when you are facing an HIS implementation. All of the manual systems currently in place to protect the privacy rights and expectations of your patients and staff do not always succeed in protecting information. Every hospital knows the problems of paper chart access: They are left on desk tops, in wheelchairs, at bedsides. They can be read by just about anyone who is literate and the least bit capable of discerning the overall organization of the record. Because of this, and because of the nature of human curiosity, legal suits have arisen against hospitals for breach of confidentiality when, for instance, an AIDS diagnosis becomes public knowledge.

Placing all of this information in a central databank does not simplify the problem; rather, it compounds it in all of the ways already discussed, plus a few others as well. Consider the implications of readily accessible isolation listings, easily cross-referenced source-of-payment notations, do-not-resuscitate orders, marital status listings and other personal information. The possibilities are as endless as the ensuing problems such possibilities create. Nothing that creates potential is without potential difficulties as well.

The creation of a centralized database is the dream of many administrators—"I'll finally be able to find out"—and the list ranks from "real" mortality rates to monthly infection rates on a per physician basis. The bottom line in all of this is that once it is in computerized database, it's accessible—by anyone with sufficient incentive and enough computer savvy to bypass the routine system controls and security levels. I recently used a system that assessed my security level, decided I was getting into information it deemed beyond my clearance, and admonished me with a cryptic, "Your access to this data is being recorded." It did not prevent my access, however. In addition, I was prompted by the message to ask who looks at the record of who recorded what. I was not terribly surprised to find the answer was, "no one." Certainly audit trails are interesting, but they do not cure the ill of unauthorized access; nor do they guarantee that anyone is ever checking the audit reports to see who is looking at what. And this does not even touch the issue of piracy-level access.

The corporate world has long dealt with the problems of unauthorized access by forces external to the corporation. This type of access is something no hospital is really prepared to deal with. Prior to electronic databases, access was simply a matter of running the gauntlet of the routine medical records department chart request services, no mean feat in most instances—and an effective deterrent as well. In the future, hospitals may face the choice of allowing access via computer terminal rather than through manual reproduction of the record; requests may be for fax reproduction via phone lines from the computerized database. There are increasing demands being made by everyone from government offices to third-party payers for data access. Requests that we now pay rote acknowledgment to when servicing them may cause us to raise our collective electronic eyebrows in the future as the potential for disaster begins to hit home.

It is a point worth noting that many states have Peer Review Protection Acts that shield certain classes of data from legal discovery requests. Some of the scenarios mentioned elsewhere in this chapter regarding unauthorized access would likely be easily defeated in the courts under the protection these statutes afford internal documents used for physician credentialling, disciplinary, and reappointment processes. This does not address unauthorized access that is not offered for in-court evidence, however. As previously noted, it does not take a lot of imagination to see that easily compiled statistics could speed the litigious clients' requests for more appropriate and legally obtainable information to assist their case. Clearly, the whole area of security is one that will require high-level attention and scrutiny as hospitals move into computerization of their records.

CONCLUSIONS

Bedside computers offer nearly limitless potential in terms of giving the practitioner immediate access to information and easy data entry capabilities. Because of these benefits, they are increasingly the option of choice by hospitals seeking to computerize. The considerations offered herein are simply that—considerations to be weighed in the balance of purchase decisions. The benefits these types of systems offer to the health-care industry are far outweighed by the uncertainties created by the new technology. Hospitals have always been on the forefront of embracing new technology for patient care, and bedside computers are simply the next logical step. They are a definitively usable way to standardize records and ease the pangs of paperwork so that the staff can get to the real business at hand: taking care of the patient.

REFERENCE

Carter, Kim (1985). Information system security top priority for medical records, *Modern Healthcare*, November 22.

5

Bedside Computers in the Intensive Care Unit

Arthur St. Andre and Susan Eckert

This chapter focuses on the development of bedside computer systems in the intensive care unit (ICU). Most of these systems are interfaced to monitoring equipment. This is what distinguishes them from the other types of systems discussed in this book.

By its very nature, the ICU—with its acutely ill patients, high-tech medical equipment, and high staff-to-patient ratio—is a rich source of data from both the supply and demand point of view. No other hospital department or division can equal the data demands of the ICU, in which information overload is a daily reality. Where else in the hospital are there so much data, so many people needing access to that data in order to care for critically ill patients, and so little time to spend on data analysis?

Our experience with an ICU bedside computer system began in 1982, when we installed one terminal in one ICU with a staff with no prior experience in computers. In the ensuing years, the ICU care at our 871 bed tertiary care institution has grown to three ICUs with a bed capacity of 36. These three ICUs, which account for over 10,000 bed days each year, now include a bedside terminal at each bed that interfaces with 37 bedside hemodynamic monitors, pulmonary arterial blood gas machines, and concomitant ventilators. Although our primary responsibilities are patient care, ICU administration, and professional education, we have been intimately involved in the development and implementation of a computerized ICU database entitled "QS." Produced by Quantitative Medicine, Inc. in Annapolis, Maryland, this database brought us to the point in which the capability of our current system was overwhelmed, although only 30% of the available data is computerized. Since our early hardware and software limited our growing capabilities for computerization, we have sought and received funding to replace our technological resources with a new, upgraded system.

The process of progresing from one ICU terminal to an extensive system has been filled with many frustrations and stresses for a staff faced with a high level of daily demands. Unlike many university medical centers or institutions with large endowments, we did not have the resources to devote personnel exclusively to our computerization program. In that sense, we are like many of you. By offering practical advice based on our clinical experience, we hope to help you avoid some of the pitfalls and growing pains we experienced in the early years of our computer system.

DESIGN CONSIDERATIONS

In its most simple form, a computer-based clinical data management system consists of hardware, software, connecting cables, and people who make the project work. In the ICU, the ultimate objectives of such a system are to eliminate paper, reduce clerical functions, improve patient care, satisfy regulatory requirements, and improve the overall efficiency of the unit. In our experience, we have seen many of these benefits in improved care, smoother bed utilization, and more effective management of our ICU. The expectation that any computer system will satisfy all of those objectives is, however, unrealistic, particularly in the misconception that reductions in personnel will be a natural by-product.

Nevertheless, there are special design considerations for ICU systems that can enhance the system's productivity, ease of use, costs, and overall integration into the ICU setting. Such considerations must incorporate the wealth of information involved in the care of acutely ill patients. The depth and breadth of such data range from activities of daily living and medications to urine output and sophisticated hemodynamics. Each piece of data, with its potential importance to the data base, represents a challenge to those staff responsible for storing the data. That challenge involves not only capturing all the appropriate clinical data, but also scrupulously editing those data for accuracy before storage.

FACTORS TO CONSIDER

Speed of Data Entry

Any system used in the ICU setting must be capable of speed, growth, and flexibility. The goal of the system should be data entry with the fewest keystrokes and programmed analysis. The software–hardware configuration must be inherently quick, with the goal of 1 second between striking the return key and mimicking the next keystroke. The user should be allowed to type ahead of the screen-echo of the keystrokes.

With ICU data, the numeric keypad is heavily relied upon for entering long series of numbers in a short period of time. For this type of data entry, light pens, mice or touch screen are not particularly useful since they essentially preclude typing ahead of the screen. They are useful for other types of data such as breath sounds, which could be satisfactorily entered with a pointing device.

There are other features that can enhance rapid data entry. These include the following:

1. Designing a screen that contains many data elements in one frame. This allows the user to make multiple entries without changing the screen.

2. Promoting rapid navigation from one data point to another. An efficient system will allow the user to move data elements at the top to the middle and back again without excessive use of the return key. An indexing scheme or skip rule moving automatically to the next point can be extremely helpful.

3. Permitting the echoing of prior data elements en masse to the most recent entry. This feature is especially helpful for patients with a systems exam such as neurology which is unchanged.

4. Keeping data elements that have been or are about to be entered in sight throughout the entry session.

5. Using table-driven menus that automatically appear on the screen when the cursor rests on the pertinent data. For example, if the element is cardiac rhythm, the menu provide an automatic selection such as a) atrial fibrillation, b) atrial flutter, c) premature atrial contraction, d) premature ventricular contraction, etc.

6. Using automatic signals for elements infrequently entered but necessary. For example, if cardiac rhythm is ventricularly paced, all the elements necessary for documenting pacing variables appear in a window.

Security

Concerns about the security of an ICU database must balance principles of "reasonable protection" with the avoidance of extremes in user identification. One extreme, for example, would be a system that forces the recording of a user identification and password with each single element. The other extreme would be a permissive system in a unit with a rotating pool of staff and no system for identifying one-time users.

The best security system requires all users to label data they are responsible for recording, while also allowing for data entry in a series of recordings such as all the respiratory settings. There should also be a system of data editing that requires users to sign on at the beginning of a shift, to be confirmed as a user during the shift, and to be manually signed off at the shift's end.

Data Entry Accuracy

Any clinical data monitoring system must be configured with editing procedures that ensure a high degree of accuracy and reliability. Although it is virtually impossible for a system to recognize all user errors, there are editing parameters that can be useful in maintaining high-quality data. These parameters include the following:

1. *Ranges for physiologic possibility and probability*: Similar to parameters used in laboratory-based systems, these ranges designate the acceptable scope of a particular data element. Any score outside of this range

is automatically rejected, forcing the user to recheck the figure. Data values that are within the realm of possibility but not probable should generate a query for the user to confirm the value. If the user confirms the value with the "yes" key, the number is accepted. For example, a heart rate of 30, which is possible but not usual, should generate an editing message.

2. *Variables assessing anatomic and physiological compatibility*: These more sophisticated editing procedures serve as second-level backup systems for anatomic and physiologic compatibility. Anatomical edits check the appropriateness of sequential data. For example, a user who records right leg strength in a patient with a documented right leg amputation would be queried. Similarly, a user would be queried after entering a physiologic variable that was not compatible with other related data entries. For example, it is not possible to have a PCPW of 18 with a pulmonary artery mean or artery diastolic of 10.

3. *Delta checking for repeat variables*: This type of edit compares sequential data for the same variable. If a change in a physiological variable is improbable, the system issues a query. Examples might be a systolic blood pressure that rises from 100 to 250 in an hour, or a blood urea nitrogen (BUN) level that rises from 10 to 50 in 6 hours.

Similar types of editing checks can also be used with descriptive data such as the physical exam, although these data are more difficult to screen. For example, a query would be generated if a user entered wheezing and no breath sounds in the right lower lobe for the same patient. The data could represent a transcription error or two clinicians recording the same type of finding in a different way.

System Configuration

Any ICU system must be capable of growth in size and expansion in terms of complexity. The system must have the flexibility to enable the users to add, subtract, and edit their data elements and flowsheet configuration.

To achieve the optimal configuration scheme, vendors and the ICU staff must work together to develop a system with the optimal performing capacity required for the needs of their ICU. Such collaboration will provide opportunities for the ICU staff to participate in the development of their own computerized system. The specialized expertise of the ICU staff can be utilized in answering important questions involved in the configuration and reconfiguration of an institutional system. For example, the data set for the physical exam requires knowledge of factors such as the following:

1. Components that are necessary for monitoring actual care and those that must be documented for regulatory purposes
2. Medical terminology that most accurately represents the specific end point, i.e., describing the degree of muscle strength vs. the degree of muscle weakness
3. The reasonable and necessary descriptors of patient care
4. Terms used for describing the physical exam which will keep interrelator variability to a minimum, i.e., describing the size of the pupils in millimeters or as normal, small, or large). Requirements for patient care as well as early warning signs must both be considered.
5. Use of global term vs. specific indicators such as "pulse check" or a specific prompt for the dorsalis pedis

An additional issue with system configuration is determining the sequence of data presentation. Some systems provide a configuration scheme in which the data are presented in a sequence resembling a clinician's thinking vs. the sequence in which data were entered into the system.

The task of configuring a system is a complex one, requiring input from key individuals and caution in avoiding unnecessary complexities and information overload.

Issues Related to Time

In ICU computer systems, the time of recording information presents a number of questions and potential dilemmas. Consider the number of "times" for any particular data element—the time of data recording or the time of reporting (i.e., in laboratory services). In addition to reporting these real times, there are instrument times for physiologic monitors.

How, then, is the "best" time recorded into the system? The answer depends on the level of specificity required to care for and monitor the patient as well as the degree of complexity involved in coordinating data from multiple sources into a reasonably chronological sequence.

Our experience has shown that the use of time windows can be a great asset in structuring data entry. For example, recording all vital signs and input/output data at scattered times throughout an hour can result in a difficult-to-interpret data display. Instead, a system configured with a time window in which the time appears over a column of data to be recorded every 10 or 15 minutes can organize the time points more efficiently, while decreasing the user interaction and the chances for error. In our system, the internal time clock advances every 10 minutes.

Data entry of time also requires editing procedures to detect errors. These may occur when the time is inadvertently recorded in the future, or if the time is recorded as "old time," or that older than an hour.

Interface with Other Data

One of the greatest benefits of using a computerized ICU system is its ability to interface with a variety of reporting systems. There are those that enter the system directly via monitoring or data-acquiring devices such as hemodynamic monitors, pulse oximeters, and intracranial pressure monitors. There are interfaces with therapeutic devices such as fluid infusion pumps and ventilators. And there are linkages to systems external to the ICU that provide results reporting such as laboratory, radiology, and noninvasive studies.

Of the current systems available on the market, physiologic monitors providing real-time output, digitized electrocardiograms, blood pressures, and cardiac output are among the most developed. Those with therapeutic devices are less developed but have significant potential in future field testing.

Most critical to the success of the ICU system is complete interface with the external results reporting system. An effective and efficient system for reporting laboratory results is essential in the ICU. An interface with the laboratory can save critical time while also eliminating great dependence on the telephone. This feature is especially important today when nursing time must be conserved for direct patient care.

Other interfaces that are being planned by vendors but are not yet available include linkages to reference data banks, statistical software packages, and other external sources of information.

Building the Database

With the wealth of data available in the ICU, how do you decide which elements receive priority entry into the new database? Our experience has shown that the database should be built in modules that can be phased into the operation over a gradual period of time. Data that are used more frequently and those most amenable to manipulation with computer power should receive priority entry into the system. These include the following:

Physical Examination

As previously discussed, a well-designed computer program can utilize the menu format for the physical exam. Data to be included are vital signs, arterial pressures, pulse, pulmonary artery pressures, central venous pressures, respiration rate and pattern, and cardiac output. Additional information from the physical exam is added for specific diagnoses. For example, intracranial pressure would be added for a patient with head trauma. Findings from a patient with asthma would include the quality of breath sounds, pulmonary secretions, etc.

Nurses Notes

This essential part of the patient's medical record can become a logical extension of the documentation of the physical exam. Nurses' notes become more condensed as the level of table-driven physical exam notes increase. Since they are necessary for the chronologic documentation of events, careful planning must be done to assure concise, consistent data entry for nursing functions. Basic nursing care and activities of daily living such as sleep time, ambulation, nasal care, bath, catheter care, and skin care are easily coupled with the physical exam data.

More difficult decisions arise from translating the traditional SOAP format into the computerized system. For example, do assessments remain a component of the chronological note or become part of the significant events sections, or the problem list, or all three? Such decisions are best made collaboratively with the clinical staff responsible for data entry.

Test Results

As previously mentioned, the results of tests from laboratory and radiology services are essential components of the database. These data should be added to the system in its germinal phase because they contribute so much to the care of the patient and to saving clinician time.

Admitting, Discharge, Diagnosis Data

These data, while not essential to patient care, are cornerstones of the administration and utilization of the ICU. Although these data are simple to enter, they change frequently along with the working diagnosis and complications.

Intake/Output Data

These data are good examples of balancing the computer's benefits, i.e., tabulated I/O totals versus the disadvantages, i.e., the labor involved in recording each constituent and the volume infused each hour.

Physician Orders

There are two distinct advantages to incorporating all physicians' orders into the database. First, such orders can be linked with the interfaces in the pharmacy, central supply, etc. Orders are then quickly, clearly, and concisely transmitted, thus saving time, paperwork, and transcription errors. Second, compliance with physicians' orders can be checked frequently to assure a high level of control and quality assurance.

The disadvantage is, of course, that such entry requires an increased use of the system by physicians, which may be met with some resistance by the medical staff. Our experience in actively involving the staff in the development and implementation of an ICU system is discussed in the following section.

OPERATIONAL ISSUES

As previously stated, a computerized clinical database is composed of software, hardware, connecting cables, and the people who make the project work. Without the willingness of the staff to use the system and their active involvement in system development and refinement, even the most sophisticated system will fail. The key role of staff is central to the operation of the system.

The adjustment of medical staff to computers has been reported in the literature throughout the past 10 years. The phenomenon of computer resistance (Gibson and Rose, 1986) has been widely identified and may be related, in part, to a lack of familiarity and understanding of the operations and practical applications of the technology (Grobe, 1984). Fears about job security (i.e., will machines replace personnel) reliability, loss of crucial patient information, and the system's complexity contribute to staff uncertainty about the usefulness of a computerized system.

There have been a variety of studies that have explored nurse's attitudes about computers. Stronge and Brodt (1985) and Krampf and Robinson (1984) developed instruments to measure attitudes toward computerization and potential areas of resistance. Research has shown that individuals in their mid 30s and younger adapt more quickly to computers than those over 50, whereas there was no significant difference in attitudes when users were compared by educational level or prior computer use.

In one survey, the majority of nurses believed that computers would enhance patient care, increase their personal satisfaction, and improve productivity (Krampf and Robinson, 1984). In another study, Bongartz (1988) compared two groups of nurses: users of a hospital information system that included nursing care plans and nonusers employed in a hospital with no computerization. Results from this study demonstrated more positive attitudes towards computers by the nonuser group in the areas of the computer reducing paperwork and saving time that could be used on direct patient care. No difference was found between groups with issues involving the potential legal ramifications of using a computer system, the willingness to use computers, or the other potential benefits from such a system.

The goal of the ICU management team is to not only minimize staff resistance to the system, but also invite their active participation in developing and modifying its components. Our experiences in organizing and analyzing the data and, at the same time, ensure that our system is user friendly have presented constant challenges. Through trial and error, we have learned some valuable lessons, which are presented below in a series of steps that can be followed during implementation of an ICU computer system.

1. *Identify a key player.* Organizational support for the computer system will not, in and of itself, ensure the success of the system unless there is an individual involved in the selection process (from its inception) to the daily operation in the clinical area. This person should have the authority to develop and implement policy and have clinical responsibilities and a long-term commitment to the organization. This individual must be computer literate so that he or she can adequately assess the system's ability to handle the data needs. Rotating the responsibility for selection, implementation, and modification of the system can lead to decreased productivity as the new individuals suffer through the "learning curve" associated with a new project. The key player in our organization has been instrumental in acquiring, developing, and upgrading our clinical information system in conjunction with individuals from the hospital information systems division, biomedical engineering departments, clinical staff, and management personnel.

2. *Utilize the appropriate personnel.* Selecting the system is an awesome task and responsibility that is complicated by the fact that many existing systems have been tested only in smaller organizations that are not as complex as the ICU data. The literature provides some insights into staff resistance, but little practical information on systems development. In reality, this means that selecting a system is an internal decision.

At our institution, we utilized an interdisciplinary approach involving the medical director of our ICUs, the chief of biomedical engineering, a clinical ICU nurse specialist, and several members of the hospital information systems division. We have actively solicited clinical user feedback from nurses via demonstration sessions that allow an introduction to a particular system. When evaluating this type of feedback, remember that perceptions of a system's capabilities can be limited by experience and knowledge. For example, when we were selecting our system, the staff was enthralled with the ease of one particular system. The same system, however, could not perform the required interfaces with other departments such as the laboratory. Since the staff perspective is generally limited to individual needs rather than organizational needs, it must be objectively integrated into the total perspective of the project.

3. *Implementation strategies.* After a system has been selected, education becomes a priority. Initial education for all users must be planned, along with ongoing programs for new users entering the clinical area.

4. *Obligate the vendor.* In the contract with your vendor, be sure to obligate the vendor to specific staff education programs. Key issues include initial and follow-up training schedules, provision of a written training plan detailing content and timeframes, and provision of an interactive computer-based tutorial for ongoing education and training sessions for support personnel.

5. *Provide a structured orientation.* The use of a structured presentation including generic principles of computerization has been shown to positively influence nurses' attitudes towards computers (Ball, Snelbaker, and Schetner, 1985). A formal orientation with a brief introduction to the terminal and hands-on training has proved effective in introducing new staff to our computer system. The orientation, held once a month for 4 hours, is directed by a staff nurse who is a computer expert and who is comfortable with group instruction. Class size is limited to 10 or fewer with an optimal ratio of four to five students per terminal.

Remember that the user group's previous exposure to a computer system will significantly affect instructional strategies you use. Users without any exposure to a computer system will obviously require more structure and support than those with experience. In general, a brief formal presentation followed by a competency-based, self-learning module performed at the terminal will be the most cost-effective method for meeting a variety of learner's needs.

6. *Allow a gradual introduction to the system.* After the formal introduction, all users should receive guidance in utilizing the system during their unit orientation period. Preceptors reinforce concepts covered in class as they introduce functions one at a time. For example, an orientee will be shown simple procedures such as how to admit/

transfer/discharge a patient within the system and how to obtain drug calculation charts. Commonly used functions are then gradually introduced one at a time until the entire system is mastered.

7. *Develop a computer resource manual.* A resource manual that describes functions, common problems, and resolutions is an invaluable tool at the early stages of orientation. It is also helpful in assisting staff who are learning at different speeds. Houle (1980) identified the following differences in groups when adopting change. Innovators explore new ways of approaching problems/changes. Pacesetters are progressive and derive satisfaction from social interaction and from being the first to adopt innovations. The middle majority, the largest group, follow pacesetters in accepting new innovations. The laggards or "die-hards" may never adopt the change.

With these differences, there will be a period of time in which only a few staff will be able to effectively solve problems and utilize the system fully. A written manual, therefore, can be of great help for staff when experts are not available during the day shift, and for those who work nights and weekends.

8. *Identify expert users.* The innovators and pacesetters within the staff can be helpful in managing the tremendous change brought about by the computerized system. The enthusiasm and expertise of a cadre of strong clinical users can be utilized for identifying problems and potential solutions, assisting other staff, and providing feedback for future development. Management support for these users is crucial and should include paid time for the above activities, as well as paid attendance at regional computer conferences.

9. *Make the system user friendly.* Features that make an ICU system user friendly have been identified in the first section of this chapter. Here are some additional strategies that we have found helpful in overcoming staff resistance to the computer system:

   a. *Implement the system in phases.* Obviously, it would be overwhelming to initially implement an entire system. In our experience, implementing in phases (i.e., respiratory data, neurologic data, etc.) allows the staff time to become familiar with data entry and presentation, while also allowing time for assessing the system's ability to handle the volumes of data being entered and stored.

   b. *Implement desirable functions first.* Since staff are motivated to use the system when it provides tangible benefits for them, we recommend initially implementing functions with rewards. For example, one of the first features we included in our system was a very simple, but very popular calculation called the "Drip Chart." This function quickly calculates and prints the intravenous drip rate or dosage upon command. When titrating a drug such as Nipride, such a chart provides a quick reference for a variety of infusion rates.

c. *Utilize familiar terms.* Whenever possible, use terms that are routinely used. In our system, the neurologic chart contains a qualifier that pops up after the user enters the data associated with the Glasgow Coma scale. Under the category "eyes open," the qualifier chart initially read "paralysis." Although the intent was to identify patients who were under anesthesia, the item was incorrectly interpreted by the staff as one of those patients who had been administered paralytic agents. The item was then changed to read "anesthesia" with no further confusion.

d. *Input items in a familiar sequence.* Users will be more compliant with data entry if it is presented to them in the usual order. For example, an arterial blood gas is generally reported in our system in the following sequence: P_aO_2, PCO_2, pH, HCO_3, BE. Changing that sequence would cause confusion and data errors.

10. *Have a clear back-up procedure.* Although vendors assure purchasers that downtime is minimal, it can and will occur. Clear guidelines for the staff during those times will decrease the frustration associated with the system's malfunctioning. In our system, we do not require staff to reenter or catch up by entering data that was generated during the system's failure. Such double documentation only reinforces negative attitudes about the system and, in reality, is not required if adequate supplies of manual records and forms are available on the unit for such instances.

11. *Activate a unit/hospital computer committee.* Implementing an ICU computer system is a mammoth task. Although software is provided by the vendor, it must be configured to fit your organization's needs. That process is an extremely time- and labor-intensive task.

We have found a computer committee to be helpful in organizing and managing this task. Since three ICUs in our hospital are currently utilizing a computerized system, a committee with representatives from all three areas, along with others involved in its operation such as a physician, clinical specialist, respiratory therapist, and information systems representative meet monthly to review problems and plan future applications.

The clinical and administrative perspectives have been invaluable. Bedside users contribute suggestions and concerns relevant to their practice, and administrative personnel collaborate in evaluating clinicians' priorities for developing a system congruent with organizational goals. We have also formed unit-based committees for implementing suggested changes on the unit level.

This broad-based, multidisciplinary committee structure has been very effective in helping our system progress in its development.

12. *Be patient.* Any ICU computer system is complex because it is designed to manage massive amounts of information. Be patient! Implementation realistically takes place over a period of months and years. Setting long- and short-term goals can help you make that transition successfully.

REFERENCES

Ball, M., Snelbecker, G. and Schecker, S. (1985). Nurses perceptions concerning computer use before and after a computer literacy lecture, *Computers in Nursing*, Jan./Feb., 23–31.

Bongartz, C. (1988). Computer oriented patient care, *Computers in Nursing, 6*, (5), pp. 204–210.

Chang, B. (1984). Adoption of innovations: Nursing and computer use, *Computers in Nursing*, Nov./Dec., 229–235.

Gibson, S. and Rose, M. (1986). Managing computer resistance, *Computers in Nursing, 4*, (5), 201–204.

Grobe, S. (1984). Conquering computer cowardice, *Journal of Nursing Education, 23*, (6), pp. 230–239.

Houle, C. O. (1980). *Continued Learning in the Professions.* San Francisco: Jossey Bass.

Krampf, S. and Robinson, S. (1984). Managing nurses' attitudes toward computers, *Nursing Management, 13* (7), pp. 29–34.

Stronge, H. and Brodt, A. (1985). Assessment of nurse's attitudes towards computerization, *Computers in Nursing, 3* (4), pp. 154–158.

6

Nurse and Physician Perceptions

Joyce E. Johnson

This chapter presents the results of a survey that we feel reflects the perceptions of many who read this book. As was pointed out in the first chapter, not many hospitals are utilizing the bedside computer terminal concept. Therefore, many reading this book will be nonusers, who may find their views similar to those who responded to a recent survey.

Ten years ago, technological forecasters predicted that interaction with computers would be a daily routine for many workers. In health care, that prediction is slowly becoming a reality as computers become as essential as the Kardex once was in nursing stations. Indeed nursing management has welcomed the secretarial relief provided by computerized information systems which can order supplies, request and report laboratory results, organize both patient and staff scheduling, and maintain financial billing systems. But will nurses welcome or resent the presence of computers when they are used at the bedside as aids for nursing care?

Computer terminals at the bedside can provide nurses, physicians, and other hospital staff with instant access to important clinical and laboratory information. Computerized systems at the bedside have, in some hospitals, completely automated the standard patient charting system with its volume of reporting forms for nursing notes, vital signs, intake and output measurement, medication records, patient care plans, orders, laboratory results, and other financial billing forms. As such systems eliminate the paper medical record, they ultimately influence the human factors involved in the physician-nurse-patient relationship and in the delivery of care.

The recent growth of bedside computer systems, the lack of research on the impact, and their potential illustrate the pressing need to study this emerging trend in health care. The following survey, conducted from January to August 1988, and presented at the New England Healthcare Assembly in September 1988, was designed to determine the level of interest and resistance both physicians and nurses associated with the use of bedside computers and to determine nursing and physician "readiness-to-change" with the integration of new computer systems at the bedside.

DESCRIPTION OF THE SAMPLE

As outlined in Table 6.1, a total of 50 community, teaching, rural and urban hospitals located in the Mid-Atlantic and New England regions were selected and asked to respond to the nursing survey. A total of 39 (78%) hospitals responded with the majority of respondents representing small hospitals with fewer than 400 beds.

Each hospital was asked to provide survey data from five nurses, with each one representing five skill areas. A total of 181 nurses

Table 6.1. Nursing Respondents by Hospital Size

Bed Size	Number of RNs	Hospitals
0–100	18 (10%)	4 (10%)
100–200	43 (24%)	9 (23%)
200–300	48 (27%)	10 (26%)
300–400	43 (24%)	9 (23%)
400 & Over	29 (16%)	7 (18%)
Total	181	39

Source for Tables 6.1–6.3: Joyce E. Johnson and Patrick F. Abrami (1988). Bedside Computer Perception Survey.

responded, with 34 responses from ICU head nurses, 37 M/S head nurses, and 29 M/S staff nurses.

In addition, each hospital was asked to offer a general invitation for physicians to participate in the survey. As outlined in Table 6.2, a total of 52 physicians responded from 16 hospitals, with 24 (or 46%) of the respondents from larger hospitals, with at least 400 beds.

Participants in the survey were asked to respond to a variety of questions related to their perceived associations between bedside computers and factors such as productivity, technical feasibility, costs, benefits, staffing, nurse/physician/patient relationships, and paperless record concept.

Responses were measured using a Likert scale with a lower limit of one and an upper limit of four. Respondents were also asked to indicate if they believed each variable would produce the expected positive or negative response in the bedside setting.

Each of the survey questions was evaluated by individual variables with an overall numerical rate; a percentage indicating overall negative or positive response; and an analysis of the most positive responses by nursing skill areas and hospital bed size.

SURVEY RESULTS

Nursing Perceptions

Key findings from the survey showed that nurses believed that automating clinical activities such as charting, results reporting, care planning, patient assessment, order entry, and medication administration would increase their productivity. Head nurses from hospitals with 200–300 beds perceived the most benefits from automating those functions that were rated, in descending order of belief of increased productivity, from 3.61 to 3.20, respectively on the Likert scale, with 93% to 77% indicating that they felt productivity would be increased. Automation of other functions such as administration of intravenous fluids, patient scheduling, ancillary staff scheduling, and posting of charges were perceived as less related to nursing productivity with rating of 3.17 to 2.59, respectively, and 76% to 67% indicating that productivity would be increased.

Table 6.2. Physician Respondents by Hospital Size

Bed Size	Number of Physicians	Hospitals
0–200	14 (27%)	4 (25%)
200–400	14 (27%)	5 (31%)
400 & Over	24 (46%)	7 (44%)
Total	52	16

In the evaluation of adaptability to automation, staff nurses as a group felt it would be most difficult to adapt to patient assessment charting, and reporting results with computers, whereas head nurses expressed concern about adjusting to computer-based scheduling systems for patients and auxiliary staff. In the evaluation of those same functions from a standpoint of technical feasibility, head nurses continued to express a lack of confidence in scheduling systems, a response that may reflect recurrent difficulties with existing scheduling systems.

Data from the ranking of benefits from a fully operational bedside computer system show that environmental and physical benefits were perceived as the most likely benefits to be realized. These included less walking, improved accuracy and legibility of records, improved ability to retrieve data for research, and immediate availability of patient charts, with rating ranging from 3.33 to 3.14, respectively. Less realistic views were seen for the computer's effect on improving productivity, decreasing unit clerk hours of overtime from charting and hours of direct nursing care, and improving nursing morale, the ratings ranging from 2.83 to 2.44, respectively. As in previous questions, head nurses continue to optimistically view the bedside computer system as a helpful management tool.

In terms of cost and benefits of using computers, head nurses were the most optimistic about the cost of computerized systems being offset by their benefits. Seventeen percent of the nurses responding felt the cost-benefit ratio would be positive, with another 56% indicating that the computerized systems could possibly pay for themselves. The 25% of nurses who were not sure were predominately staff nurses from large hospitals with over 400 beds.

Preferences for either a hand-held or a stationary computer terminal showed, not surprisingly, that head nurses preferred stationary terminals at the nursing stations whereas staff nurses preferred a hand-held terminal that they could carry with them on the nursing unit.

In the additional section of the survey, nurses were asked about a variety of effects of bedside computers on such variables as nursing dynamics, the nursing shortage, and the patients. Over 50% of the nurses surveyed viewed bedside computers as one helpful solution to the nursing shortage. As in the previous sections, head nurses perceived the most benefit from computerized systems. The head nurses also perceived a positive effect of bedside computers on the dynamics between the physician, nurse, and patient. Head nurses in the medical surgical areas viewed the addition of computers as a very positive change because the nurses and physicians would develop a closer relationship as they both worked side by side using the computer system.

In assessing patient reaction to the system, the majority of those same head nurses from M/S units predicted that, since the computerized system presents a more organized image to patients, patient care would improve with the addition of computers at the bedside. Almost one-third of head nurses in the ICU felt that patients would have no reaction to the computers, suggesting that the patients have adjusted to technologic equipment at the bedside or that the severity of their illness decreased their sensitivity to bedside equipment.

When asked to evaluate the potential difficulty in adjusting to the paperless patient record, the majority of nurses felt they would initially feel insecure without the usual patient record. This insecurity was expressed predominantly by ICU head nurses in hospitals with 400 beds or greater. Staff nurses from M/S units in small hospitals expressed the most optimism about the adjustment period. A total of 24% of all nurses responding predicted that they would adjust quickly to the paperless record with little or no training.

Despite the nurses' overall resistance to change and concerns about the adjustment to computer, 89% of all respondents were "willing to be a pioneer" in bringing computers to the bedside. Head nurses in the M/S units were, again, the most optimistic group, whereas nursing administrators were more cautious in the willingness to adapt to the change.

Overall, the nurse respondents saw many positive effects from bringing computers to the bedside. A total of 45% saw computers as a time-saver, 32% as a convenient way to access information, 24% as a means for improving the legibility and accuracy of patient records, 21% as a means for eliminating duplication of documentation, 14% as a means for eliminating paper, and 10% as a method for standardizing the patient medical record.

On the negative side, 31% of the nursing respondents believe that the learning curve with computer literacy would be long, 18% felt a computer downtime would be a disadvantage, 15% were concerned about costs, 10% had concerns about physician acceptance and patient confidentiality, and 10% thought that computers at the bedside would increase the clerical functions nurses were asked to perform.

Physician Responses

As a group, the 52 physicians who responded to the survey also perceived considerable benefits from computers at the bedside although their perceptions differed from the nurse's perspectives.

A total of 63% viewed computers as a partial solution to the nursing shortage, compared to 84% of nurses who envisioned computers as nurse-extenders. As outlined in Table 6.3, physicians perceived the primary benefit of computers as improved accuracy and legibility of records, compared to nurses who ranked the elimination of walking as the primary benefit.

Table 6.3. Nurse/Physician Perceptions of Benefits

Benefits	Response Weight*	
	Physician	Nurse
Improved accuracy and legibility	3.21	3.17
Accessibility/eliminate walking	2.93	3.33
Efficient retrieval of data	2.81	3.15
Immediate availability of chart	2.48	3.14
Increased productivity	2.37	2.82

*On a scale of 1 to 4 in which one was the least beneficial and four the most beneficial.
Source: See Table 6.1.

Physicians expressed greater doubt about the ability of the computerized systems to pay for themselves, with 22% suggesting that the capital costs would never be recovered, compared to only 3% of the nurses who expressed concern about the financial loss from such systems. Two-thirds of the physicians, like the nurses, preferred stationary computer terminals, with one-third preferring a portable terminal. The majority of physicians surveyed viewed an office terminal as important.

In the assessment of the computer's impact on nurse/physician/patient dynamics, the physicians were slightly more concerned than the nurses about the potential negative effects, with a total of 14% of physicians versus 3% of nurses predicting a negative change. Physicians, like nurses, thought that computers would effect no reaction from patients (45% vs. 54%, respectively).

Physicians expressed greater confidence than the nurses about their adjustment to computers, with 36% predicting no problems in adjusting to a paperless patient record. Nevertheless, the physicians were less willing to change than the nurses (62% vs. 89%), and 33% suggested a "wait and see" attitude, compared to 11% of the nurses.

Overall, 22% of the physicians viewed computers as a positive influence on information retrieval, 22% noted decreased paper as a benefit, 14% saw information synthesis as a plus, and 12% saw improved accuracy and legibility as positive influences that computers would have at the bedside.

Negative comments offered by the physicians included cost (14%), downtime (12%), diminished physician/nurse interaction (10%), and increased clerical responsibility for physicians (8%).

Implications

The survey results demonstrate that both nurses and physicians perceive significant benefits to computerized patient systems at the bedside, and are willing, interested and ready to make the changes needed to incorporate such systems. Head nurses perceived the most benefits from such systems, whereas nursing administrators were the most cautious from a cost standpoint. Physicians perceived significant benefits from results reporting and data analysis. Both groups perceived increased accuracy and legibility as the primary positive outcome from computerized systems, and downtime or memory loss as their area of greatest concern.

All of these findings provide valuable insights into nursing and physician perspectives on computerized systems at the bedside. Since nurses and physicians will be the critical linkages between patients and bedside computers, more research on the integration of computers into patient care is needed.

7

Strategies for
Introducing Change
Among Care Providers

Frances R. Vlasses

The utility of new technology can only be appreciated in a work environment that is open and accepting to this technology. Management and staff join with physical, social, and cultural factors to influence the creation of this environment. An organization's unique identity is carefully imprinted in the work setting and must be understood if changes are to be successful. This chapter provides concepts useful to the understanding of this environment and presents strategies to assist in developing implementation approaches. These concepts are especially true when dealing with a change as major as implementing bedside computer terminals with a reasonable amount of functionality.

CHANGE

Introduction of automation into an organization has interesting ramifications that affect the organization at the individual, group, and community levels. Frequently, responses to automation are referred to as "computer anxiety." However, upon a closer look, computer anxiety addresses the individual's response to the computer in the case where they may never have dealt with one before. The individual may describe being anxious, being concerned they are not able to learn the necessary skills, and being worried that the computer will inhibit their privacy. However, this explanation for change response seems somewhat superficial.

It is more helpful to consider the introduction of automation into an organization and its implementation on a broader scale using broader frameworks. One helpful framework that brings to bear on this process is the notion of automation as a second-order change. Most of us are familiar with change concepts that describe change as a direct, linear process characterized by an executive order or an innovation to improve care delivery or a change related to the developmental stage of the organization. From a systems perspective, planned changes tend to occur at the outside boundaries of an organization.

Examples of this include the implementation of primary nursing or conversion to a unit-dose pharmacy system. Such examples are contained within a department, and, while they require a lot of staff work and energy, it is fairly easy to define the beginning, the middle, and the end points of these change processes. Automation and the utilization of integrated automated systems rely heavily on converting communication processes. It is important to realize that we are actually dealing with an internal organizational function and can expect much more unusual staff responses for this reason. Automating information flow from one department to another and interacting with the communications that had previously been verbal between members of the multidisciplinary team cause change impacting the fabric of the organization. In fact, second-order change is change that takes place at the interface of an organization's philosophy, professional practice, and work habits. Computerization can affect these areas. Information display communicates standards, practice, and management philosophy to staff. The fact that the computer is at the patient's bedside and at every other work station will surely affect work habits. The act of "charting" will require that documentation styles be modified and that thinking processes be adjusted to come into line with system documentation requirements.

Using an automated system at the bedside may also cause some concern about the larger societal issues. Questions may arise regarding confidentiality and intrusiveness. This type of content again reminds us of the characteristics of second-order change: that it is a root change requiring policy-making changes, that it is fairly radical in its nature, that it is, frequently, revolutionary change, and that it has nonlinear qualitative aspects. This type of change process starts in one place and then implodes on an organization causing and requiring change that was not anticipated initially. Therefore, this framework for second-order change serves to inform us of the kind of change strategies and leadership that are necessary in implementing an automated system.

Decentralized group work seems to be needed. It is the recommended approach to computer socialization and feedback. The process, however, of working with large, decentralized groups can appear very chaotic. The workload is heavy. People may discuss issues that had previously been considered sacred cows and pet peeves. Turf issues get center stage. Newness and the committee structure can be threatening to traditional management lines, and the process is one that lends itself to decision avoidance and rehashing. Frequently, rumors abound. There may be a high degree of confusion and conflict over specific tasks. These factors can be very threatening to project leadership and can, in fact, be blocks to productivity.

Recognize that the group members may be trying to learn and do at the same time. They are in a situation where they are trying to learn a new system and make decisions about its use simultaneously. This is a new role for clinical and management staff who generally have a fairly high degree of knowledge about the decisions they are called upon to make.

The natural response to this kind of group behavior is for leadership to become more controlling; to limit information flow, and to highly structured meeting time. What looks like an increase in confusion and frustration and a decrease in productivity from the outside may be symptoms of second-order change but not the disease.

The disease is the loss of control the individual experiences when confronted with work automation and how it translates to the organizational level. In fact, the individual's sense of control really reflects one's internal sense of competence. For management staff, competence is threatened by the fact that the larger group is in the process of evaluating practice as well as departmental functioning. Management traditionally likes to say, "yes," "no," "do it now." But now they find themselves in situations requiring, "I really don't know." For managers, this process is taking place when they have had little time to assimilate the system and its potential impact. Also, total information about the system's functioning may not be available to them.

The staff nurses' sense of competence is more closely tied to their practice. Staff, more than management, are probably more aware and concerned about the computer's impact on work habits.

In this kind of environment, leadership that is controlling is counterproductive. Strategies that serve to loosely hold the group, that allow for a combination of active communication and that direct the group members toward work goals are considered more productive than controlling behavior, especially in the early stages.

The goals of leadership in this process are very clearly to develop an understanding of the system so that changes can be identified and made, to get workers to identify their work habits (a very difficult task because they may be unexamined), and to continue to support traditional departmental structure so that departmental work continues.

In all cases—in the early stages of database review, in the development of training programs, and in the actual implementation process—maintaining and supporting the individual's internal sense of competence must and should be a primary concern. Project management must continually battle the computer's ability to intimidate new learners; the potential for the computer to dictate practice, and the misinterpretation of information made possible by the combination of mechanical quirks and human perceptions.

The strategies that are useful in managing this change include the use of strong leaders but not bosses. Strong leadership is necessary to define the task and the work but not the details, to be able to allow the group to do its work and not put a lid on issues prematurely, and to push the group toward resolution on issues of conflict.

Through the process, it is important to create opportunities for decision-making and for control over implementation deadlines and approaches. It is recommended that project leadership not overplan all aspects of the implementation to allow these opportunities for staff input to emerge.

Training packages that support self-learning as well as integrate opportunities to simulate real work at the bedside are also useful in supporting the individual's sense of control.

It is suggested that all individuals working on the project maintain a clinical focus. In addition, it is important to beware of the tendency toward perfectionism. An approach of trial and error is much more effective and less anxiety provoking than a perfectionist approach. Perfectionism can be the enemy of implementation.

Leadership must also know when to turn the discussions into action. The use of realistic deadlines can be highly effective in producing group movement as well as allowing opportunity for group discussion and analysis.

Management must be prepared to take risks, to trust the group, and to encourage an atmosphere of "doing it over" if it is not right the first time. A sense of humor will also help to keep the project going and lessen the tension as deadlines approach.

EXPECTATIONS OF IMPLEMENTATION

When computer systems are acquired, there is always a great deal of enthusiasm and hurry to get them operational. In reality, however, one must consider the fact that the preparation of database and staff requires an important resource: time. Implementation time lines have a great deal of impact on the quality and quantity of work that is achieved. Basically, one is probably looking at three different sections in three different phases during implementation in a nursing department.

The first phase begins with a feasibility study, the actual purchase of the system and the necessary preparation of the database. This phase can last a year or more. This period may require the highest investment in labor, and is also marked by the highest degree of uncertainty because it is in this period that people are trying to adjust to the idea that their practice will be affected by automation. It is also in this phase that all relationships and communication lines are being identified and established for implementation. These include relationships between departments and information systems, the hospital and the software vendor, all staff working on a nursing unit, and senior management and department level managers and staff. In this phase, themes emerge that will be the source of the most resistance. One can begin to see emerging leadership. Because the amount of work in this phase is very high, the use of firm deadlines can be very effective. All work can be divided and compartmentalized. Deadlines should be firm and not extend beyond 6 weeks; the work should be divided in such a way as to fit into those segments. This gives an opportunity for leadership to bring the group back together for status reports and for group members to mark progress. It is suggested that although the groups can be run democratically, the effectiveness of this phase will be determined by how well defined the work is and how well enforced the deadlines are.

The second phase usually begins with preparation for an actual installation. Frequently, this occurs on a pilot unit and is initiated with the training of staff.

Two opinions exist about the use of pilot units. One is that the pilot unit should be relatively low key, yet involve representatives of each discipline. Another approach is to use a very fast-paced unit to adequately test the system. In any case, the use of a pilot unit serves a variety of purposes. Beside the fact that it allows opportunity for testing in a real environment, it also serves to allay a lot of anxiety about whether or not the system will really work. A significant change usually occurs in the tenor of the project following actual implementation. Staff worry less about developing the perfect database and become much more reality oriented in the creation of screens and identification of problems.

Labor needs in this phase are also high, but are much more directed than in the first phase. Initially, staff training is very labor intensive because evaluation of the training package is also taking place if it is being utilized for the first time. In addition, information services staff are needed to assist in monitoring the actual pilot, and 24-hour nursing support must be a consideration depending on the level of implementation of the application.

One should decide, on implementing a pilot, whether or not it is going to be time limited and whether or not the application will remain installed following the close of the pilot. It is helpful if the unit staff participate in this decision.

Although project team members generally are responsible for designing the implementation approach, decisions, as much as possible, should be left to the unit management. The unit manager on the implementation unit is the individual who must ultimately wrestle with policy decisions that will arise with the implementations, with staff reaction, and, also, with an increased number of individuals to ensure that they are carefully educated and supported through the implementation, and it is advised that she or he be included in planning meetings as soon as the pilot unit is identified.

The second phase generally closes with the completion of the evaluation studies that are performed. Staff reaction, database and hardware performance, and educational programs should be evaluated. It is not uncommon that additional training will take place 1 month to 6 weeks following this implementation. Some of the problems that are identified may be reconciled through training, and the learning curve is such that individuals will be anxious to learn more about the computer in this context.

The third phase generally begins following the first implementation. This phase is marked by a broadening vision, especially on the part of the database developer, who looks at how the current tools will be used in other units throughout the hospital. The initial work of database developers, at this point, will be to refine the database incorporating evaluation data and to begin meeting with members of other units to identify special needs for implementation to that unit. The overall training package for the hospital should be finalized in this phase.

Problems in this phase occur if deadlines are too long and people are not able to see the results of their labors. The enthusiasm of the first two phases are gone now, so morale occasionally becomes a problem. At this point, leadership must remember that guidance and direction will be necessary to keep the project on course. However, project staff will tend to be much more realistic in terms of workload and accomplishments and can be directed to develop tools that are much more reality based than are initially considered.

It is also in the third phase that labor needs should be reconsidered. Number of staff and hours utilized in the first two phases may no longer be necessary, depending on the pace of the project, and projections can more easily be made regarding the need for full-time staff. It is recommended that full-time project assignments not be made until this phase is achieved.

THE EVALUATION OF PRACTICE

One of the most critical yet subtle aspects of implementing a computer system is the opportunity that it allows a department to evaluate their practice approaches. This aspect provides an unusual exercise that may range from reaffirming departmental practices to developing new policies.

When the database is received from a vendor, it is necessary that a user group be formed to review the clinical content as well as the data presentation in this database. This necessary part of the implementation allows clinicians to ask questions about what is really important for documentation and what is necessary to communicate to other professionals in their own discipline and in other disciplines.

Forethought must be given to the organization of this work, including the development of timelines and deadlines. It is important to utilize the principles of group dynamics in constructing and administering the work of this group. The atmosphere should support open communication and interchange of ideas. It is equally important to provide structure because this task can become overwhelming and groups will tend to get stuck on the horns of dilemmas presented by clinical issues.

Subgroups may need to be developed to address specific specialty issues. However, all information should be reported back to the larger group for careful cross-review. Special attention should be paid to the care-planning formats. Despite the fact that nurses frequently debate the usefulness of care plans, most nurses identify this aspect of the nursing process as important to their discipline and will want to insure that the format presented on the computer meets their philosophical expectations and departmental goals.

The work of this group should further be directed to topics such as formats for assessing patients and what theoretical frameworks are included in these assessments, care-planning design and style, the handling of abbreviations, and determination of whether or not information is displayed to other disciplines in meaningful format.

Information discussions with other disciplines may be in order, especially in areas of overlap such as psychosocial assessments and medication administration. Hopefully, information services staff are involved at this point, are aware of how database is being developed in each discipline, and are evaluating for major discrepancies and inconsistencies.

This group will need a great deal of encouragement to resist fixing everything that has ever been wrong with documentation.

DEVELOPING A USER GROUP

It is common to utilize a user group to do the major work in implementing systems. These formats allow for staff participation and help to socialize the organization to the issue of automation. The members of this group receive some status in the organization and, frequently, a great deal of stimulation.

These groups should be constructed very carefully. It is encouraged that the chief nursing executive and the top nursing management team participate in choosing members of this group and that these people be formally appointed by the department. The department gives this project priority and support by allowing necessary time for participation in these meetings.

Because the computer system should adequately represent practice formats and should enhance the functioning of the clinicians, it is suggested that expert clinicians be involved in the development of the database. These individuals should be very familiar with the actual delivery of care, and it is recommended that they be first-line care providers as opposed to specialty consultants. Specialty experts, management staff, and continuing education staff should participate in this group, but the majority should be representatives of the first-line clinical roles.

Each member must realize the responsibility and the time commitment necessary to complete this project. It is also suggested that these members continue to work in the clinical arena so that they continually have an opportunity to apply and evaluate their new learning as well as to formulate thoughts on issues and recommendations for the automated system.

By clearly identifying and communicating the charge of the user group internally and organizationally, the nursing department leadership can provide the philosophical cornerstones to guide participants and project leadership. This group must be sufficiently empowered to insure that their recommendations are followed.

Have no doubt that automation will raise issues regarding practice and care delivery. Having access to guiding principles will provide direction for participants as they make decisions and reclarify their thinking regarding nursing practice in an automated environment. Once identified, these guiding principles, communicated through the charge to the user group participants, can be a powerful management tool to insure that the project stays on course with departmental goals. Although each department will have to identify its own agenda, three suggested inclusions are described: control of practice, individuality versus standardization, and amount of change.

COMPUTER VERSUS CLINICIAN CONTROL OVER PRACTICE

Clinicians are concerned that automation requires relinquishment of control, especially in the practice arena. This is probably one of the most threatening issues that confronts the clinician when faced with automation. User-group members should receive a clear message that their job is to insure the clinician's control over practice. This principle set down, the development of this group and the reinforcement of this principle can serve as a very powerful source for cohesion and provide momentum to keep this project progressing. Nurses invited to work on this project should know that they were chosen because of their clinical expertise and that the computer should recognize and support that expertise as opposed to being in conflict with it.

Standardization Versus Individualization

The department should also be clear on the amount of uniformity or individuality it will allow and support. Because computers are fairly nonforgiving, standardized approaches are easy to support. However, decentralized management structures combined with specialized units make for high levels of individuality in nursing practice units. One can expect that without reaching good consensus, there will be much resistance to standardization in a highly decentralized environment.

This may be seen as a restriction of practice. The department needs to be very clear on how much individuality it will support in documentation. This issue continually comes up in the development of selection screens and in the attempt to make systems user friendly.

Automated Solutions

The second issue of consideration relates to the tendency to have the computer fix every problem. The department must be very clear about why the system was bought and what it attempts to accomplish by it. Members of the user group must be reminded about whether they are trying to automate a documentation system that already exists or whether they are creating a totally new documentation system. It is suggested that, because of the amount of change staff must deal with in automation, that one try to implement only one change at a time. The change to automation is intense. It is wise to match the automation system with the documentation system that already exists so that nurses are not dealing with a totally new documentation style as well as a computer. The user group will have to be continually reminded of these principles. It is suggested that management clearly outline these topics as well as others that may be important for their department.

When choosing members for this group, it is important that one think carefully about a variety of characteristics. Because deadlines are frequently intense and the work can be fairly demanding, group members should be able to work under pressure. One should look for members who are secure in their role and who can be articulate in group settings. They should be individuals who can deal with a fair amount of flexibility and who have the ability to think ahead and hypothesize what might be. It is not necessary and it is not recommended that all members of this group be committed to automation. In fact, there is some value in having the most resistant members of the department participate in this project so that they can evaluate and have some control over how the system affects their practice.

Frequently, the most deviant members of the group are the ones who have the most creative ideas for solving the dilemmas that will arise in this process. One should consider having adequate representation from each unit in the hospital. It would be necessary to represent each specialty as well as each type of worker. A member should be selected who represents the Quality Assurance Department.

The first meeting of this group should allow for introductions from all people who will be impacting the work of this group. Vendor representatives and members from Information Services should be chosen to meet with this group, and to provide liaison and continuity. Early in the work of this group, it is suggested that they identify the issues of major concern. These issues can provide the format of the early stages of work, and give project managers and department heads an idea of what the thorniest issues will be.

This group needs to have good access to the department's policies and procedures, and to be well aware of how the department operationalizes these policies. Many hospitals, before actually receiving their database, go through a process of revising policies and procedures, updating and revising them so that they are current and accurate for computer implementation. There is usually also an expectation that new policies be developed by this group. Because of this, it is important that the reporting mechanism from this group to management be clearly defined.

The Integrated Progress Note

The actual progress note is an area for special attention in automation. The definition of the progress note, in any institution, is important before automation can take place. It is also important to know who needs to see what data, when, where, why, and how. The progress note has basically the patient's response to treatment and the plan of care as defined by each clinical domain. It is important information to be shared among the caregivers. However, in the process of creating an on-line integrated chart, more issues evolve relating to the computer's ability to compartmentalize information and display it differently. The relative importance of specific clinical information differs among the disciplines. Also, the computer's ability to collect data once and use it over in different formats quickly raises turf issues. This issue really defines the possibilities of integrated systems. However, this is fairly futuristic for the state of interdisciplinary practice. What in fact is called "integrated documentation" in manual charts is chronologic charting in progress notes by a variety of disciplines. This area is source for the most excitement and possibility for patient care in terms of improved clinical decision-making and possible time savings.

COMMUNICATION

A chart is a communication tool, a vehicle by which all members of the interdisciplinary team talk to each other about the patient. In addition, progress notes reflect our values about patient care and frequently reflect our theoretical frameworks. For this reason, we see different kinds of charting systems in place. Some may be built around problem identification lists, some may be built around general systems review, some may include nursing diagnosis.

Whatever the choice, it is clear that progress notes and chart format is very influential in showing how department's values and expectations are operationalized. In addition, individual writers have their own style and charting systems are also designed to meet expectations of the reader. These readers may be as diverse as different kinds of specialists, department heads, quality assurance, and medical records personnel. So it is clear that although the chart is basically a communication tool about the patient, it is also very much influenced by the expectations of the larger community of hospital staff.

In addition, the chart presents a very special symbol in the hospital culture. There is a communication that occurs, sometimes nonverbally, around the patient chart by which the nurse knows when orders are written and sometimes knows when the physician has visited the patient. The act of order writing frequently triggers a communication process by which patient-care needs are communicated to other departments in the hospital. In this regard, the chart plays a vital link in the organizational communication process. For these reasons, computerization, in general, and computerization at the bedside can be expected to play a major role in the way an organization operates since the computer will affect the speed and the style of data presentation. What a computer does that is different from what a chart can do is that, to some degree, it can talk back, it can sort, and it can allow for structure and uniformity, which can decrease individuality. It can present an organization or a department's values in a way that can be restricting. The technology available to transmit messages, order entry, patient schedules, and chart review can have major impact on the way information is received and multidisciplinary caregivers communicate with each other, or can lessen the need for that communication. The communication issue, then, becomes an important one to evaluate in the implementation process because of the impact on patient care and hospital function. One should be concerned about maintaining the integrity of communication processes until new, natural links are formed.

Implementing a bedside terminal provides many opportunities for a type of discussion and evaluation to take place at an interdisciplinary level. This allows an opportunity to increase awareness and strengthen communication among interdisciplinary providers. It should be expected, however, that these sessions will also provide an opportunity for providers to scrutinize each other's practice domain in the way that may not have been anticipated. For this reason, it is suggested that interdisciplinary meetings to review database and screen development be handled with caution. As a general rule, it is suggested that each discipline be fairly secure with their database before it is released for review in a meeting format.

A great deal of attention should be paid to the communication processes and styles used for implementation because the computer does affect the communication processes of the caregivers. It is important to have regularly scheduled meetings where any interested member can attend to discuss the status of the project. It is important to provide feedback sessions where individuals are encouraged to report complaints. Access to project management and hospital administration is important at critical times throughout the project and should be expected. Daily meetings should be expected during the actual implementation for fast problem identification and solution. Also, it is useful during actual implementation to develop an evaluation sheet that can be placed at every terminal to identify problems quickly.

Following the initial implementation, it is important to maintain communication with new users. Frequent rounds on the unit are suggested. Also, as the computer database is evolving and improving, users will also be interested in knowing how the database is improving and what is happening in other departments. Many institutions are using newsletters to handle this kind of information.

Be forewarned that downtime is best handled by advanced communication as well as follow up communication for problem identification.

TRAINING

The training package is frequently expected to address all staff needs including their resistances and their values about automation as well as to raise their competency level. In designing a training package, one must carefully sort out these expectations with an eye to realism. The issues of resistance and the socialization of the users should be dealt with early in the project. It is unwise to wait until training begins to deal with those issues. In fact, the inclusion of staff early in the project can be a very powerful strategy to engage resistant staff. Consciousness-raising activities can take place from the beginning of the project to encourage acceptability. In-services demonstrating the system, newsletters, and progress reports to staff are all techniques that can be used to encourage support and socialization.

The actual training package should be defined in the first phase of the project and can be a source for staff input. It is expected that the computer literacy level of the staff will be quite diverse. For this reason, it is recommended that staff training programs be developed to allow time for new users and also be developed in such a way that experienced users can progress with self learning directives. Three-hour training sessions tend to be most effective. A high percentage of hands-on experience should be allowed to encourage competency. Also, some attention needs to be paid to the differences between using the computer at a desk and using the computer at the patient's bedside. This can be addressed by discussion groups and on unit training, which is necessary to ease the transition to using the computer in the clinical area.

General guidelines for the training program include the utilization of a short demonstration session; to allow the learner to go on the system and do return demonstrations and then to provide an educational experience with them that they can progress through at their own pace.

It is suggested that trainers be carefully chosen. Individuals with patience and ability to handle resistance and difficult questions should be sought. Many hospitals utilize on-unit trainers who are identified and brought together for the total hospital implementation. These individuals also serve as contact people to provide training updates as system changes occur.

It is also recommended that more than one training approach be utilized. Most hospitals will work on implementing a classroom-based training package. But in today's current health-care environment, with staffing shortages, float pools, and temporary agencies being used to a high degree, it is necessary to come up with alternate approaches to education. Therefore, alternate plans should include the utilization of unit-based inservicing as well as audiovisual (A/V) assisted training programs for use in different environments.

It is truly a challenge for the educational staff to support the pace of a computer installation project. It should be expected that the actual installation plan will change direction considerably due to multiple delays that commonly occur in a project of this magnitude.

LABOR NEEDS

Labor needs will change depending on the phases of the project. Initially, in creating a heterogeneous group, it would be important to include people who may later assume leadership roles. It is strongly recommended that nurses on the project team be very strong clinicians. Although it is difficult to find clinical people who may want to commit time to automation, some people will do it in an effort to control practice and also as an opportunity for growth. Parttime participation on the computer project is also an alternative, and may enhance clinical application of the system.

Project team members should be expected to participate in all aspects of the project including database modification training, the development of training, and staff support during implementation.

The project team should always include a group of nurses representing various job functions and clinical specialties. High flexibility, creativity, a decreased need for control, a collapsible organizational structure, and the ability to work with ambiguity are characteristics that will enhance the effectiveness of the project team. They should function under a clear dictum to create a database acceptable to clinical staff nurses and supportive of departmental standards. These guidelines will be amenable to implementation goals and will lessen the natural temptation to fix it all with the computer.

Information services staff are important to the effectiveness of the implementation. The relationship with information services should be collegial and collaborative. It is helpful to identify one nursing liaison system analyst to be a contact person and a communication point for nursing. However, at times in the project, it may be necessary to include more members of the information services staff to support the implementation. It is suggested that information services staff be aware of hospital functioning and respectful of the clinician's outlook. This will serve to decrease conflict and precipitate fewer control issues.

Vendor personnel are also on site as the project evolves. This group of staff, of course, are initially most knowledgeable about the product and its intended use. A fair amount of negotiation generally takes place between the user and the vendor, especially in the area of modification. A balance must be achieved between the vendor's intended use and the practitioner's actual use. Sometimes these negotiations can be very stormy and will need third-party intervention. In many cases, however, product enhancement can occur through these discussions.

For many staff nurses, this may be the first time that they have had the opportunity to work within a committee structure as well as interact with members of nonclinical disciplines. Support and encouragement need to be offered to members of the user group by nursing leadership to encourage their participation and to assist them in developing the necessary communication skills to be effective in this setting.

8

Designing and Conducting Benefits Evaluations: An Analysis of Three Hospitals

Louis E. Freund

The first questions asked by those considering installation of a bedside system regard the system's projected benefits. How will the system affect the efficiency and effectiveness of patient care? How will recovery of the system's costs be achieved and when will the recovery be completed? Will the documented and perceived benefits be sufficient to generate acceptance on the part of the clinical staff who will be expected to integrate the system into their daily routines?

Benefit analysis is concerned with the above questions, and others as well. Among these are the following: How will the system affect the quality of patient care and the quality of nursing care? Will the system provide the patient with a higher degree of confidence or satisfaction about the care process? Will the effectiveness of ancillary services be increased, and will patient outcomes be improved?

Clearly, then, the potential scope of benefits evaluations is very broad, touching on every area of management and clinical concern. However, any evaluation is in some way limited to some level of available evaluation resources and time. Real world benefits evaluations must therefore be designed to focus on those features of organizational and clinical processes that are most impacted by the system's structure and most important to the philosophy and goals of the organization.

At the same time, benefits evaluations are usually conducted in unusually charged settings which include new techniques and technologies, the normal stresses of patient care responsibility, and the presence of ad hoc measurement methodologies and personnel. Studies must be designed and conducted to assure the validity and impartiality of the results. Otherwise, the entire effort may generate more confusion than it resolves.

This chapter presents an approach to designing and conducting benefits analyses that includes subjective and objective measurement methods. As examples, a series of three studies of a specific bedside system are presented in detail.

DESIGNING THE BENEFITS EVALUATION

The premise of this chapter is that the purpose of a benefits evaluation is to objectively determine the overall contribution of the bedside terminal system to the organization's productivity. This means that we wish to determine how the system has impacted the quantity and/ or quality of services provided to the hospital's patients and medical staff, and the degree to which the bedside system may have impacted other systems and procedures within the hospital. As a result, a thorough understanding of the bedside system's impact on methods and procedures becomes the foundation for evaluation study design.

Methods documentation provides two important components of the benefits evaluation study:

1. The documentation highlights aspects of the manual operation which will be different following implementation, and becomes a guide for the possible utilization of different benefit studies.

2. The methods documentation becomes the formal system definition for all benefits observed and attributed to the system under study. Since systems are usually being upgraded and modified, any benefits study represents the system as a specific level or

status in the system's development. The methods documentation establishes a formal description of the system's status as of the time that the benefits evaluation was carried out.

Methods documentation, in the form of process charts, should be undertaken for each major activity or function that the system impacts. The documentation results will highlight differences between pre- and postimplementation methods.

But, in addition to pointing out areas of difference, the process charts will also be useful for highlighting potential areas of study. If benefits (or negative benefits) have occurred as a result of installation of the system, they are likely to be associated with the differences between pre- and postimplementation methods. These differences become the focus for specification and design of the evaluation studies.

Two types of studies are necessary to establish a comprehensive picture of the benefits of the bedside terminal system. The first type includes studies which are designed to establish the differences in time required to perform patient care functions which can be attributed to the system. Work sampling, time study, predetermined motion time systems, and other objective methodologies are appropriate for this benefit measurement requirement.

The second group of studies are designed to obtain objective measures of qualitative performance factors. These include the timeliness of data capture and recording, error rates, delays and waiting time, waste, attitudes and acceptance, rework, frequency of deviations from specified procedure, and others.

The functions performed by the system, as well as available resources for design and conduct of the studies will influence the specific approach taken. Key considerations for study definition and design include the following:

1. *Objective*: Data collection should be accomplished by third party independent observers or from analysis of routine records created during the normal course of activities.

2. *Accurate*: Data collection designs should assure that all data analyzed was accurate when recorded. Independent observers, with no other responsibilities than data collection, help to achieve this goal.

3. *Nonintrusive*: Data collection protocols should not affect the processes which are being studied. For example, studies should not re-

quire the staff being studied to perform additional tasks which are not normally a part of their jobs.

4. *Representative*: Data collection should be conducted so as to reasonably represent each shift, weekdays, weekends, and each skill level.

5. *Anchored*: Staffing levels, patient acuity, census, and other work load related factors should also be monitored during data collection in order to improve the possibility that studies will be correctly interpreted.

6. *Structured*: Data collection for each study should be accomplished according to written procedures that are provided to each observer during formal observer training. Situations that are encountered during data collection that were not anticipated by the procedures should be resolved and communicated to each other observer for that study.

An example of the application of these concepts is presented in the following sections of this chapter.

EXAMPLE BENEFITS EVALUATION STUDIES

In May, 1987, MECON was selected by CliniCom Incorporated to objectively assess the benefits of the CliniCare Point-of-Care System at three new installation sites. The studies focused on the activities of nursing and pharmacy personnel before and after implementation of the system. They included work sampling of nursing personnel activities, time study of video tape records of nursing procedures, observations of medication administration activities, interview, questionnaires, and other data collection procedures.

The results described in this chapter are representative of different release levels of the CliniCare software and implementation processes which were matched to each of the hospital's needs. Since these CliniCare System modules are being enhanced continually as a result of on-site evaluations and experiences, the conclusions contained in this chapter may only be associated with the specific versions of the software and hardware installed at the time of the various post-studies. In addition, the CliniView attachment, a 24-line multiplied by 80-character touch panel screen, was not available or evaluated in any of the studies reported in this chapter.

The purpose of these studies was to ascertain the benefits, both quantitative and qualitative, realized by each study hospital due to the installation of the CliniCare System. More specifically, the study was commissioned to:

Measure the time, activities [and] risks associated with [patient care procedures], before and after installation of the CliniCare System on a quantitative and qualitative basis including, but not limited to staff hours [or full-time equivalents (FTEs)] to perform the following tasks:

- Medication Administration and Control
- Charting Data
- Staff/Patient ID
- Controlled Substance Inventory
- Pharmacy Support
- Data Retrieval

The term "benefits", as interpreted by both CliniCare and the Hospitals, refers to demonstrations of increased productivity on the part of the Hospital's organization. Each party was interested in determining the extent to which the CliniCare System provided benefits in all areas, including but not limited to saving time, reducing risks, or improving productivity in any one of a number of additional ways. As a design philosophy, then, this study assessed the impact of CliniCare on a number of aspects of the productivity concept.

1. *Increased time with patients*: It was expected that CliniCare would cause Nursing personnel to spend more time in the presence of patients due to the additional requirements for data entry on the bedside terminal. This was perceived to be a positive potential effect of CliniCare.

2. *Improved accuracy of medication administration and I/O records*: In addition, the timeliness of chart entries for all related documentation was expected to be improved. Chart documents, graphs, etc., were expected to be more accurate.

3. *Improved procedures anticipated*: Writing and rewriting data was eliminated for the three tasks, and the chart documents recording results were expected to be more readable.

4. *Reduced cost*: The costs of providing nursing care were expected to be reduced. In this regard, the Hospital's expected reduced expen-

ditures, such as lower overtime cost, agency cost, and recruiting costs. In addition, productivity improvements for staff would generate savings equivalent to expended monies to hiring additional personnel in each skill level.

The first study site, referred to in this chapter as Hospital A, is a 311-bed Midwestern facility with 14 nursing stations. It services over 11,000 inpatients and 130,000 outpatients per year. The evaluation studies in Hospital A were conducted on a 36-bed cardiac step-down unit.

The second study site, Hospital B, is a 459-bed Southeastern private hospital. The studies were conducted on two medical/surgical units on the same floor, and results were combined across the two units.

Hospital C, the third study site, is a 159-bed West Coast facility. The studies at Hospital C were conducted on a second floor Surgical Unit.

MECON implemented a pre/postinstallation data collection design to determine the benefits which could be attributed to the three applications included in the evaluation.

The prestudies were conducted over a 10-day period just prior to system implementation at each hospital. Usually, implementation occurred in stages, with vital signs and I/O beginning first, and medication administration and medication scheduling starting somewhat later. The post studies were conducted during 10 days about 4 weeks following completion of all installation and training activities.

Methods Documentation

Methods used by nursing personnel prior to and after installation of the System for medication administation, vital signs, and I/O responsibilities were documented. Additional tasks required due to the presence of the system were noted (such as removing reports from the printer and inserting them into charts), as were tasks which were no longer required (such as adding up the I/O totals each shift and each 24 hours).

Preinstallation procedures were substantially different between the three study hospitals. Hospital A, before CliniCare, had no computer support for the medication administration function; CliniCare was implemented just after the installation of a Pharmakon Pharmacy management system. As a result, Hospital A's procedures and methods related to medication administration changed from manual to fully automated between the pre- and post-study periods. The nursing staff at Hospital A had not previously been required to routinely validate a computerized medication order database against physician orders in the patient's charts.

Hospitals B and C each had already installed pharmacy management modules as components of their medical information systems: Baxter in the case of Hospital B and SMS at Hospital C. Medication database validation was already a routine part of nursing procedures at Hospitals B and C before CliniCare was installed. Therefore, the modifications required in nursing procedures related to CliniCare functions were not as significant at Hospitals B and C. Further, at Hospital C, an automated interface between SMS and CliniCare substantially reduced the need for separate auditing of the CliniCare database.

At all study sites, several manual record keeping tasks were eliminated, such as totaling of I/O's and copying scheduled medication administration times onto a scrap of paper (referred to as the nurse's "scrap" or "brain") each shift by each nurse.

Specified postimplementation methods were well adhered to at Hospital A in MECON's opinion. However, at Hospitals B and C, it was observed that the prescribed methods were not fully implemented during the post study data collection period. "Scraps" were still being used occasionally to temporarily record data taken in the patient rooms. Also, at each Hospital, the medical scheduling function was set up with a one hour "window" on each side of the scheduled administration time, thereby relating the focus on medication administration timing errors.

MECON's study design for establishing pre- and postimplementation medication administration error rates was based on a methodology reported by Barker and McConnell (1984). The protocol required a pharmacist-observer to accompany nurses, selected at random, and witness the preparation and administration of individual doses. The observations in the pre- and post-studies were made over 60 hours, spread across the day and evening shifts during peak medication administration times. In addition, a review and comparison of the medication administration record against the physician's orders was done to identify transcription errors, prior to each observation period.

Medication Error Rate Study

CliniCare's design emphasizes the accuracy and timeliness of medication administration.

Medication error rates were calculated as the frequency of medication errors during the observation periods, divided by the total opportunities for error. Types of errors included in the studies were as follows:

- Omission
- Wrong dose
- Wrong drug
- Wrong patient
- Unordered drugs
- Wrong time
- Transcription errors

A pharmacist-observer was oriented to the study project in general, and specifically to the Barker methodology. The pharmacist was instructed, when a nurse was making a medication error, to intervene only if the error was life threatening to the patient. The pharmacist, who was not a hospital employee, was introduced to the appropriate nursing personnel on the study units and was oriented to the unit and the medication procedures.

Staff nurses were told that a medication administration study was being conducted; however, they were not specifically told that they were being observed to determine the type and number of medication errors being made.

The accuracy of medication administration improved at all study hospitals within 4 weeks of system start-up (Table 8.1). At Hospitals A and B, nursing's errors of omission and commission were virtually eliminated. At Hospital C, it was determined that a large proportion of the observed post-implementation error rate was due to orders that had never been entered into CliniCare. Stricter adherence to database validation procedures at Hospital C was expected to lower this error rate in the future.

Pre-implementation results indicated that from 15% to 25% of scheduled medications are given more than 1/2 case hour before or

Table 8.1. Medication Administration Error Rate Results

Type of Error	HOSPITAL A		HOSPITAL B		HOSPITAL C	
	% Pre	% Post	% Pre	% Post	% Pre	% Post
Wrong Dose	0.76	-0-	1.12	-0-	0.68	1.32
Extra Dose	-0-	-0-	-0-	-0-	1.82	-0-
Omission	0.76	-0-	0.84	0.92	7.50	4.23
Unordered Administration	1.52	-0-	0.84	-0-	-0-	-0-
Other	5.82	-0-	3.36	0.31	0.91	-0-
Subtotal:	8.86	0.0	6.16	1.23	10.91	5.55
Wrong Time	25.06	13.69	25.49	22.32	15.00	9.52
Total Error Rate:	33.96	13.69	31.65	23.55	25.91	15.17
Total Number of Administration Observed:	395	292	440	378	357	327

more than 1/2 case hour after the scheduled administration time. Clini-Care has the capability of noting each time errors of this type occur and listing, by nurse and patient, the frequency of such timing errors. To avoid this citation, and to avoid the extra keyboard entries required to chart the late or early med, nurses are encouraged to administer the ordered meds within one half hour of the scheduled time.

This "feature" became a problem in the actual implementation of CliniCare. The one half hour policy window significantly affected the ways in which nursing staff were able to organize their work. As a result, the computerized window was extended to one hour on either side of the scheduled time. No change was made in hospital policy, however; it remained 1/2 hour. Each hospital planned to reduce the window to 1/2 hour overtime.

In spite of the relaxation of the CliniCare time of administration "window" to one hour, timing errors in the post studies were still counted at the one-half hour window level. At Hospital A, timing errors were reduced by nearly 50%. At Hospital B, the reduction was about 30%. It should be pointed out that a modest level of early or late medication administration is to be expected, given the fact that patients are not always available or able to receive medication within one-half hour of the scheduled administration time.

The transcription error rate improved slightly at Hospitals B and C (Table 8.2). Hospital A experienced the largest improvement in this

Table 8.2. Error Rate Results MAR Transcription: Medication Administration Record (MAR)

Type of Error	HOSPITAL A		HOSPITAL B		HOSPITAL C	
	% Pre	% Post	% Pre	% Post	% Pre	% Post
No indication	5.18	2.76	1.37	1.22	3.28	4.13
No strength	1.57	0.24	0.46	0.54	0.26	0.29
No frequency	3.45	1.92	-0-	-0-	0.92	0.44
No route	0.94	-0-	0.61	0.68	6.95	3.69
No quantity	-0-	0.12	-0-	-0-	-0-	0.15
Drug transcribed wrong	0.47	0.24	-0-	-0-	-0-	-0-
Other	3.77	2.04	2.13	1.09	1.31	1.33
Total MAR Transcription Error Rate	15.38%	7.32%	4.57%	3.53%	12.71%	10.03%
Tot No. of MARs Reviewed	637	832	656	736	763	678

area, a 50% reduction in errors, probably partially due to implementation of audit protocols related to managing the new computerized medication database.

MECON concludes that the accuracy of medication administration can be expected to improve further as staff gain familiarity with CliniCare and become more confident in its design.

Interviews with Hospital Personnel

MECON conducted structured interviews with personnel at all levels of the organization during the pre- and post study periods. In general, across all three study sites, the results showed fundamental similarities. The opinions of the respondents were optimistic and apprehensive prior to installation. At the time of the post study, respondents reported positive opinions regarding CliniCare's impact on patient care and a very positive opinion about the potential for other benefits from the system in the future. The Appendix beginning on page 137 presents pre- and post-study interview results.

Additional positive opinions were expressed regarding CliniCare's ability to improve the accuracy of records, improve the ease of reviewing data at the bedside, make the nurse's job more interesting, and improve the accuracy and timeliness of medication administration.

A majority of respondents were also positive about CliniCare's contribution to making the nurse's job easier, enabling the staff to provide higher quality patient care and provide better service to physicians.

The strongest disagreement was expressed with regard to the current and eventual use of CliniCare by the medical staff. Respondents felt during the post study that CliniCare (as defined by its current set of three applications) is not likely to be a tool that physicians will use.

On the whole, a majority of respondents stated positive or very positive attitudes about CliniCare during the post study and felt that it helped address some of the Hospital's important problems.

Comparison of these results to a pre study results for the same questions is also informative. In general, respondents have not yet observed all of the benefits they anticipated. This is particularly evident with regard to the affects of CliniCare on nursing roles, physician roles, and overall feelings.

However, it is also apparent that CliniCare has outperformed expectations with regard to the observed range of benefits. A much broader variety of observed benefits emerged during the post study than was mentioned in the prestudy.

Allocation of Nursing Time

It was expected that the CliniCare System would directly influence how nurses spend their time, and several hypotheses regarding the expected impact of CliniCare on nursing time were formulated. After the implementation of CliniCare, nursing personnel, excluding ward secretaries, were expected to be observed spending:

- More time in direct patient care activities at the patient's bedside
- More time administering medications at the patient's bedside
- Less time in charting and other indirect patient care activities associated with medication administration, I/O's, and vital signs
- Less time walking between patients' rooms and the nursing station

- Some moderate amount of time in training, problem solving, and other new activities directly related to the presence of the Clini-Care System

As a result of these changes in the allocation of nursing time, it was anticipated that overtime and other premium cost resource hours would decrease. In addition, it was expected that there would be an increase in time spent in patient care that, otherwise, could have only been achieved by adding nursing hours per patient day

An objective observational time measurement technique, work sampling, was selected to study how the CliniCare System impacted the percent of time unit personnel spent in their activity categories of interest. Two work sampling studies were conducted at each hospital. The first study took place over a 10-day period before CliniCare was implemented. The 10-day follow-up or post study took place some four to six weeks after CliniCare was installed.

Data collection was accomplished by RN observers who made continuous rounds of the entire physical area of the nursing unit. As they proceeded along their randomly chosen route during one of these rounds, they made an instantaneous observation of each staff member at the moment that person was first seen on that round.

The observer recorded the skill level of the person observed and categorized the activity the staff member was engaged in at the moment of the observation. The observer then continued on the tour until after staff members had been observed or had been accounted for. Then, a random spot to start the next tour was selected. The observer moved to that spot and started the next tour immediately. The time to complete a tour ranged from 3–7 minutes, depending on the number of staff being observed.

A mark-sense data collection form was designed to allow for observation and coding of 45 distinct nursing activities. The observer could record all of the data collected during a tour on one side of the form. The categories of activity defined were based on CliniCare functionality (i.e., I/O, vital signs, and medication administration) and the anticipated benefits associated with CliniCare.

Both the pre- and poststudies at each hospital included all three shifts and three weekend days. Normally, a total of 10–20 nurses were hired as observers and trained by MECON for each study at each hospital.

Approximately 20,000 observations were obtained during each pre- and poststudy. MECON determined that this volume of data was required to assure that a high confidence level could be obtained regarding the results related to infrequently occurring activities and to provide sufficient data to obtain meaningful results by skill level.

Prior to conducting these studies, MECON projected that professional nursing time at the bedside would increase. This result was expected due to the fact that many indirect care tasks which had formerly required writing in the patient's chart (at the nursing station) would, post-implementation, be accomplished using the hand-held terminal in the patient's room. Hospital clients viewed the increased presence of the professional nursing staff at the patient's bedside to be a significant benefit of CliniCare. Results confirmed this expectation at one of the three hospital sites.

At Hospital A, which "transitioned" from manual to computerized medication administration, vital signs, and I/O procedures, net RN time at the bedside decreased by 1.6%. LPN results at Hospital A were similar. Also, it was observed that the average patient acuity points (or workload) per nurse during the poststudy was 11% higher than during the prestudy.

In analyzing this situation, MECON referred to previously published research regarding the relationship between patient care workloads and the amount of time spent in various activity categories by nursing personnel (Freund and Maukscha, 1975). It was observed that higher acuity workload per nurse, when the workload is above optimal levels, has been shown to result in less direct patient care time on the part of professional staff. Based on this observation, MECON projected that, without CliniCom, the net decrease in direct patient care time at Hospital A would have been in the range of 2% to 3%. That is, direct, or bedside care, at Hospital A would have been expected to be 0.4 to 1.4% *less*, if CliniCare had not been present.

At Hospital B, the pre- and poststudies were conducted 1 year apart, due to unanticipated delays in implementation tasks. During that interval, in addition to implementation of CliniCare, significant policy and organizational changes had occurred on the study units. For example, medication responsibilities on the day shift were transferred from RN to LPN personnel. In addition, there were many more staff hours present during the poststudy than during the prestudy: nearly 37% more hours across both study units across all shifts. This resulted in a reduction in the workload per nurse of 22% on the day shift, 33% on the evening shift, and nearly 5% on the night shift during the poststudy. Finally, Hospital B substantially modified the mix of staff between the study periods.

Direct care time at Hospital B was observed to be less than 20% for RNs during both study periods. In the context of the factors mentioned above, this result, to which MECON ascribes a high level of confidence from a statistical point of view, was not considered interpretable for purposes of this investigation. Of course, other work sampling results related to Hospital B, discussed below, are subject to the same considerations and concerns.

The studies at Hospital C yielded direct patient-care results that were fully consistent with expectations. At Hospital C, there was no difference between study periods in the acuity workload per nurse, or in any other factor, except the presence of CliniCare.

Direct (bedside) RN nursing care time at Hospital C increased by 1.6% following implemenation (from 26.3% to 27.9%). Some significant differences which can be observed within this change are increases of 1.71% to record and review medications at the bedside and 1.23% to record and review I/O's at the bedside.

Similarly, LPN bedside care time increased by just over 1%, from 29.2% preimplementation to 30.3% postimplementation. The most important increases for LPN bedside care time were 1.50% to record and review medications and 1.06% to record and review I/O's. Other, non-CliniCare-related bedside care decreased for LPNs by 1.22%.

There was no change in the proportion of time aides spent at the bedside at Hospital C: 53.5% pre- and postimplementation. Most significant among these aide results is the increase of 10.7% of the time spent recording and reviewing vital signs at the bedside and the concurrent decrease of 14.4% in the time spent at the bedside performing non-CliniCare-related activities.

The work sampling studies disclosed that there were savings in time attributable to CliniCare in the indirect care category of nursing activity as well as in the proportion of time nurses spent traveling between the nursing station and patient rooms. Further savings will be available when the use of the "brains" is eliminated as a temporary record keeping device. Use of the CliniCare terminal and other new CliniCare related tasks increased nursing workload by a modest amount. The net results for each skill level at each of the study hospitals is summarized in Table 8.3. A summary of the analysis associated with each category in the table is presented below.

1. Indirect Care Activities: Indirect care is the set of activities that take place away from the patient's presence, but which are components of the clinical responsibility of the nurse.

The studies confirm that CliniCare causes the amount of time spent by RNs in indirect care activities to be reduced. Principal causes of the reduction are the elimination of manual charting of medications administered, the elimination of manual I/O totaling, and the elimination of the need to construct temperature plots on the chart's graphic sheets. Some additional CliniCare database validation and report insertion tasks were included in this category of analysis, yielding an average net savings at each hospital 2.9% for RNs, and 3.4% for LPNs.

Table 8.3. Summary of Work Sampling Results

	RN's Hospitals*		
	A	B	C
1. Indirect Care Activities	−3.8%	−2.1%	−2.8%
2. Order Database Validation	—	—	+1.9%
3. Use CliniCare Terminal	+1.3%	+0.7%	+0.8%
4. Walking-Pt. Rm/Nursing Stat.	−2.2%	−1.6%	−3.5%
5. Other CliniCare Tasks	+0.5%	+0.2%	+0.3%
6. Eliminate Use of Scraps	—	−1.7%	−1.5%
Total	−4.2%	−4.5%	−4.7%

	LPN's Hospitals		
	A	B	C
1. Indirect Care Activities	+2.4%	−10.0%	−2.6%
2. Order Database Validation	—	—	+2.4%
3. Use CliniCare Terminal	+0.5%	—	+1.4%
4. Walking-Pt. Rm/Nursing Stat.	−4.4%	− 0.4%	−1.9%
5. Other CliniCare Tasks	+0.5%	+ 0.1%	+0.3%
6. Eliminate Use of Scraps	—	− 6.5%	−1.2%
Total	−1.0%	−16.0%	−1.6%

*Percentage change in workload.

2. Order Database Validation: At Hospital A, which transitioned from manual to computerized medication scheduling on the study unit, database validation tasks were considered to be productivity gains on the part of nursing staff and the time required for the activity was not charged to CliniCare. In other words, this was not viewed as a new task added by CliniCare, but as a long-standing responsibility of nursing personnel which had been unfulfilled until CliniCare made it mandatory.

Hospital B had already implemented such medication order validation procedures with the installation of the Baxter Pharmacy System. Little additional manual work (less than 1% of RN time) was devoted to additional validation steps during the poststudy, and it was anticipated that this validation would disappear once an on-line transfer of order data was established between the Baxter systems and the CliniCare system. As a result, no long-range projection for additional database validation tasks was included in the results summary for Hospital B.

A similar projection could have been made for the SMS system at Hospital C; however, the proportion of time spent by nurses in database validation there was somewhat higher than at Hospital B. The observed time spent in this activity which was additional to the database validation activity already ongoing to support the SMS pharmacy module was included in the summary for Hospital C.

3. Use of the CliniCare Terminal: Nurses at each study hospital performed some CliniCare terminal tasks that were not required of them before CliniCare was installed. These included such activities as requesting reports, entering patient care assignments each shift, and entering some information regarding patient care. The tasks averaged about 1% of RN time and 0.1% of LPN time.

4. Walking Between Patient Rooms and the Nursing Station: Three categories of walking were studied. In each of the study hospitals, RNs were observed to be walking less between patient rooms and the nursing station while they were shown to be walking more in both of the other categories. This reduction in travel time was expected, and the result was taken to be a benefit of CliniCare. On the average, RNs spent 2.4% less time in this category of corridor travel. The average LPN result was a reduction of about 2%.

MECON noted that there was an increase of 0.4% of LPN time in this travel category at Hospital B. (This increase is included in the above average value for LPNs.) On evaluation, this increase was considered to be the next effect of the benefits of CliniCare implementation (as observed at the other two study sites), and the concurrent addition of medication administration responsibilities to the role of the LPN at Hospital B on the day shift.

5. Other CliniCare Related Tasks: Training activity, problem solving related to the use of CliniCare, and several other tasks that were new were observed during the poststudies. The total time averaged about 0.3% for RNs and LPNs and was expected to decrease as familiarity with CliniCare increased.

6. Eliminate Use of "Scraps": As noted above, nursing personnel at Hospitals B and C were frequently observed to be recording data on scraps of paper, rather than using the hand-held units in the patient's room. The elimination of this practice is absolutely feasible with CliniCare and the result will be a further time savings. In addition, transcription errors which are inherent in the scraps to chart (or terminal) process can be eliminated at these hospitals in the future.

Pharmacy Studies

At each study hospital, implementation of the CliniCare System included modification of several procedures in the Pharmacy Department. These modifications impacted many aspects of pharmacy activity, including crediting, charging, labeling, intravenous preparation, packaging equipment, and supplies. In each case, a MECON review team, including a management engineer and a pharmacist, thoroughly documented each change, assessing the annualized amount of additional costs or savings which would accrue. Results indicated that costs and savings would nearly offset each other at two of the three hospital sites. A substantial annualized savings was projected at Hospital A. A significant part of this savings estimate was attributable to expected reductions in wanted pre-mixed fluids, due to more timely notifications to the pharmacy. These results are shown in Table 8.4.

Benefits Summary

The average dollar benefit across all three study hospitals was $386,000 per year. Total dollar benefits projected for each study hospital were as shown in Table 8.5. In addition, the system signifi-

Table 8.4. Annual Estimated Pharmacy Savings (Cost) Results

	Hospital		
	A	**B**	**C**
Pre-Packaging		$ 12,663	
Bar Code Labelling			
Labor			$(23,425)
Equipment	$(31,392)	(36.405)	(2,400)
Supplies			(328)
Order Entry			(6,302)
Dose Dispensing	40,027		(1,714)
Medication Delivery			(792)
Charging/Crediting	10,976	15,536	20,056
Research Denied Claims			174
Inventory Holding	14,100		(264)
Reduced Lost Charges		(3,300)	11,394
Implementation (Amortized)			(3,975)
Denied Claims		16,714	
Total Annual Pharmacy Savings (Costs)	$ 33,711	$ 5,208	$ 6,598

Table 8.5. Summary of Annual Dollar Benefits Projections For Total Hospital CliniCom Installation

	Projected Annual Benefit		
	Hospital A	**Hospital B**	**Hospital C**
Department of Nursing			
Reduced RN overtime charges			$ 78,345
Reduced agency fees			124,938
RN productivity increase			
equivalent to	$271,608	$224,182	38,628
LPN productivity increase			
equivalent to	9,868	329,979	4,922
Aide productivity increase			
equivalent to			5,110
Subtotal:	$281,476	$554,161	$251,943
Forms Elimination			7,646
Incident Report Processing Time			1,121
Pharmacy Net Annual Savings:	$ 33,711	$ 5,208	($ 6,598)
Reduced Reimbursement Denials	$ 31,868		
Total Projected Annual Benefits:	$347,055	$559,369	$254,142

cantly reduced medication administration errors, and improved the timeliness of medication administration. MECON's studies also determined that significant transcription error rates, computational error rates, and delay in recording I/O and vital signs data in patient charts were eliminated by the system.

REFERENCES

Barker, K. N., Harris, J. A., Webster, D. B., et al. (1984). Consultant evaluation of a hospital medication system: analysis of the existing system, *American Journal of Hospital Pharmacy*, 41.

Freund, L. E., and Mauksch, I. (1975, June). Optimal nursing assignments based on difficulty, USPHS 1-R18-HS01391.

9

The Nursing Shortage: Is Technology the Answer?

Mark S. Gross, Joyce E. Johnson, and Lillian K. Gibbons

Although advanced computer technology has already provided the nursing profession with some powerful tools for managing information, its potential as a palliative solution for the nursing shortage remains unproven. Health-care information systems are valuable assets in decision making, record keeping, scheduling, and budgeting, but can they really stretch the reach of an already short-handed nursing staff?

In December 1988, the first report of the Secretary's Commission on Nursing answered that question in the affirmative. Established in December 1987, by Secretary of Health and Human Services Otis R. Bowen, M.D., the 25-member commission found that although no single solution could solve the national nursing shortage, nursing information system (NIS) had the potential for conserving nursing time spent directly on patient care.

The commission had been given a one-year mandate to assess the nature and extent of the nursing shortage; identify successful recruitment and retention practices; and to recommend short- and long-term strategies for resolving the pressing issues in nursing today. After a year of regional public hearings and research, the commission identified this shortage as demand driven and proposed a system of efforts for enhancing nursing recruitment and retention in the private and public sectors. As outlined here, utilization of nursing resources was a primary area of concern in which the potential for NIS would come under the Commission's scrutiny.

Secretary's Commission on nursing categories of recommendations:

- Utilization of nursing resources
- Nurse compensation
- Health care financing
- Nurse decision making
- Development of nursing resources
- Maintenance of nursing resources

SAVING AND STRETCHING LABOR WITH INFORMATION SYSTEMS: THE COMMISSION'S RESPONSE

In addition to creating innovative staffing patterns that recognize education, experience, and competence, the commission's report called for the development of systems which conserved nursing time for the direct care of patients. The commission found that information technology could yield impressive results not only for the nursing profession, but also for hospitals and the health-care industry at large.

Systems such as those that automate the documentation of patient care can transform data into organized, useful information. The transformation can improve the quality and cost-effectiveness of patient care as well as the morale of those rendering care. Although not yet fully proven, information systems, said the commission, hold much promise in providing practical labor-saving solutions.

Several key issues in today's health-care industry underscore such potential. First, economic issues such as cost containment require efficient and effective ways to process information. Second, improvements in the productivity of health-care professionals are directly linked to the financial bottom line of health-care institutions. Third, external regulatory pressures are demanding quality care at a reduced cost. Fourth, and finally, the business environment of health care today gives the competitive advantage to those organizations that can define, measure, and document a better quality of care. These organizations then use their competitive edge to attract more patients and maintain a highly qualified staff.

All of these issues revolve around obtaining accurate, complete, and timely information—the type made possible by computerized information systems designed to meet the needs of contemporary health care. In the past, information processing in health-care organizations relied on data processing to record, process, and track primarily financial transactions such as the billing and collection of payments from Medicare after it was introduced in 1965. In the 1970s, the health-care managers used such systems for generating and reporting revenues. The 1980s, with the advent of diagnostic related group (DRGs), the prospective payment system, and the Tax Equity and Fiscal Responsibility Act broadened information needs in health care from billing systems to the sophisticated analysis of case mix, results reporting, patient care systems, and productivity.

The 1990s, however, will focus on financial survival and delivery of quality care. Health-care managers will need advanced information systems to aid in making difficult decisions for maintaining profit, defining and measuring quality of care, and attracting and retaining skilled personnel. That need prompted the Secretary's Commission to recommend that health-care executives should expedite and broaden the use of health information systems within their organizations. Systems focused on nursing services must be an integral part of such efforts, the commission concluded.

HEALTH CARE INFORMATION SYSTEMS: BENEFITS AND COSTS

Within the health care environment, health-care information systems (HCIS) can be applied to three major areas in which different benefits can be realized from their use. Task support systems are those, as the term implies, that assist health care professionals in conducting routine procedures such as accounting; admission and registration; ordering materials, laboratory, pharmacy, and special procedures; and maintaining centralized, automated patient medical records. These systems enhance the speed, accuracy, and staff time required for information transmissal and retrieval.

Decision support systems provide analytic support for health care managers who must make critical decisions about financial issues, case management, diagnosis assessment, quality of care, product line management and professional performance. These systems organize large quantities of data into a format which can be analyzed for trends or specific indicators of performance.

Competition support systems offer managers valuable tools for defining and maintaining their share of the health care market, in an ever increasing competitive environment. These systems have the potential to define provider and payor network profiles, management health maintenance organization (HMO) and preferred provider organization (PPO) contracts, obtain patient referrals, and assist in bidding for third party contracts.

The cost factors associated with implementing these types of systems facilitate appropriate design and include costs for acquisition, software and personnel. Initial acquisition costs include proper sizing of hardware including terminals and printers; set-up charges; consultation fees for defining the required memory and disc capacities; and maintenance charges. Software costs include consultation fees for matching the right software with the needs of the organization; acquiring and maintaining the software; and defining the staffing requirements needed to support the software package. The Commission believes that the bulk of costs could be spread across the entire hospital indirectly, if all could agree to the patient care information piece of the system; individual institution needs could be tailored beyond the basic approach. Personnel costs revolve around developing career paths which will attract quality staff; providing the appropriate staff training and education; and planning for the inevitable turnover of key personnel. Costs related to facilities design involve construction or remodeling of appropriate sites to house the computer systems as well as the development of a security and disaster recovery plan to protect both the facilities and the investment in computer equipment, as well as sensitive patient data.

All of this investment in time, money, and resources can reap multiple benefits for health care organization. When properly implemented, HCIS can identify and control costs while increasing worker productivity and job satisfaction. In addition, HCIS can improve levels of service, decision making, cash flow, and the overall quality of information used by health-care executives to support quality patient care. The extent to which these benefits are realized is directly dependent upon the care with which the organization has planned and implemented the automation process. Thus, the benefits of automation are not automatic and can only be fully realized with careful, strategic, and tactical planning.

Health Care Information Systems: Nursing Applications

HCIS can be applied in nursing in a variety of ways and have significant potential benefits for nursing, patients, and hospitals. These applications are:

- Patient assessment and classification
- Care planning
- Charting and documentation
- Quality assurance
- Discharge planning
- Staffing and scheduling
- Clinical nursing decisions
- Nursing management decisions
- Point of care systems

NIS, which are gradually becoming accepted in nursing stations, have been used successfully as tools for both patient assessment and patient classification according to severity of illness and level of dependence. In addition, NIS programs and tracks nursing costs associated with DRGs.

Automation with NIS reduces the paperwork and transcription errors associated with traditional charting and documentation systems. Efficient staffing scheduling can also be facilitated with NIS. Nursing management decisions can be enhanced by tracking acuity, cost and productivity. And, with computer terminal at the bedside, in examination rooms, and in patient homes, NIS can incorporate a point of care capability through which data entry and retrieval can be accomplished with speed and without duplication of effort.

TECHNOLOGY AND THE NURSING SHORTAGE:
THE INDUSTRY REPLY

The incompletely explored potential for the many applications of information systems in nursing led the Secretary's Commission on Nursing to seek advice from vendors in the computer industry. On May 9, 1988, the commission invited a sample of vendors to testify on how information technology could be used to alleviate the nursing shortage. These vendors included Baxter Health Care, CliniCom Inc., CritiKon Incorporated, Health Data Sciences Corporation, IBM Corporation, Micro Healthsystems, Inc., SMS Corporation, and TDS (formerly Technicon).

Testimony from these industry leaders consistently supported the hypothesis that technology could be a very positive effect on the nursing shortage. The vendors cited four areas in which there was a direct positive correlation between technological system in hospitals and the ability of nurses to deliver quality care with a less-than-ideal staff/patient ratio.

First, according to the vendors, nursing productivity could be improved by automating nursing care plans, progress notes and documentation, and the entry of orders into patient charts. Automation could, therefore, help nurses complete the essential "paperwork" in much less time, time that could be better spent with the nurse at the patient bedside.

Second, the vendors indicated that the quality of nursing care could be improved as timely, and complete data relevant to nursing decisions were readily available. Technology can provide a common clinical database and can eliminate inefficiency in data management providing nursing agrees to a taxonomy that can link nursing care to the larger data set of health care and outcome of care. Nursing practices and outcomes need to be developed.

Third, the reduced clerical work, increased time available for direct patient care, and improved team spirit that result from automation translate into increased job satisfaction for nurses. And for nursing administrators faced with increasing demand for nurses, increased job satisfaction becomes a key factor in retaining staff and reducing nursing turnover.

Fourth, the vendors also indicated that these benefits from NIS could be realized in a cost-effective way to stretch nursing services. Ultimately, the institution could achieve benefits from improved nursing recruitment and retention and a considerable return on their investment.

Nursing information systems are dollars well spent:

- More accurate, accessible data
- Improved productivity
- Enhanced communication
- Decreased turnover
- Reduced labor costs

Return on Investments: Case Studies

The commission on nursing asked the computer vendors to substantiate such claims with data from hospital-based case studies that analyzed the costs and benefits of NIS. The vendors cited a variety of studies which documented savings in nursing labor, decreased turnover, and improved nursing productivity. Among these case studies was a hospital that implemented a new patient care system and conducted a benefits realization study (Tadaro, 1988). Key findings from this study showed a reduced response time for accessing patient information and test results, reduced telephone calls by nurses, and enhanced nurse-to-nurse and nurse-to-physician communications. The hospital reportedly saved $375,000 during the first year, and projected a savings of $950,000 in the second year and $1.7 million annually thereafter.

Another hospital with 511 beds implemented a computerized system with bedside terminals (Childs, 1988). Results from this cost-benefit study demonstrated a saving of 45 minutes to two hours per shift, elimination of overtime caused by late charting, and a projected savings that would offset the cost of the system in 4.7 years.

In another study, a bedside terminal system was implemented in a nursing unit with 14 nurses (Micro Healthsystems 1988). Follow-up studies showed that intangible savings were $57,000 annually as a result of reduced charting time. Tangible savings amounted to $259,000 annually through reductions in nursing overtime. The nursing department projected a saving of $301,000 from not having to fill budgeted, full-time equivalent nursing positions. In total, the hospital projected a $1.5 million benefit over the first 5 years of computerization.

Still another study of a bedside terminal system was conducted by an independent insurance carrier to examine input/output and vital sign documentation and medical administration procedures (Childs, 1988). The key finding from this study was that nursing labor savings provided a 21.4% return on investment during the first 5 years of computerization.

One 460-bed hospital implemented a new patient care system and conducted an internal review of its benefits (TDS, 1988). The hospital reportedly saved 1.2 nursing hours per day, while realizing a 20% savings in the nursing budget and a sharply reduced nursing turnover rate that was 100% below the national average.

Another similar study was conducted in a 300-bed hospital which implemented a patient care system (TDS, 1988). In this study, computerization resulted in a work force reduction of 39 FTE positions over a 2-year period, a figure that was 70% of the hospital's original projection. The hospital also reported that nursing turnover was 76% below the national average after the NIS was implemented.

Finally, the vendors cited a study in which a 200 bed hospital implemented a new patient care system and later achieved estimated productivity improvements of 10–15% of its nursing personnel (TDS, 1988).

TECHNOLOGY AND THE NURSING SHORTAGE: THE NURSING PERSPECTIVE

After hearing such positive responses from the vendors, the Secretary's Commission on Nursing then focused its attention on assessing the nursing perspective on technology at the bedside. To do so, the commission conducted a telephone survey of 10 of the 30 nursing administrators who currently have point-of-care systems operating in their hospitals, in either a test environment or fully operational.

The results of this survey echoed the responses from the computer vendors. The nursing administrators identified many advantages to NIS: improved productivity in nurses and other hospital personnel as well; elimination of overtime for charting; improved morale; improved compliance to documentation standards; easy accessibility of chart data; decreased medication errors; and decreased use of nursing personnel from temporary agencies.

The nurses emphasized that although improved productivity does not necessarily reduce the need for nursing FTEs, it does "open the door" for restructuring staffing patterns, overall redesign of the workplace, and improvement in new methods of operations.

The difficulties with using NIS said the administrators were focused on operational issues such as limited software; lack of integration of the systems with the hospital as a whole unit; difficulty training the float personnel; logistical difficulties in placing terminals in appropriate locations in patient rooms and nursing stations; and the slow response from vendors in enhancing their products to meet the perceived needs of their organization.

Nursing administrators cited five key factors which were critical to the successful implementation of NIS:

- Comprehensive planning
- Phased implementation
- Management support
- Appropriate software
- Adaptable software

The basic issue, concluded the nurses, is that the success of NIS is directly related to the nurses' initial perception of the long-term benefits of such systems. The most successful use of NIS was found in those nursing divisions which, through careful planning and implementation, made the systems work for the mutual benefit of the patients, nursing staff, management, and the hospital as a whole.

THE COMMISSION'S CHARGES: TO HEALTH CARE EXECUTIVE AND VENDORS

All of the expert testimony and the Commission's year-long research led to the same recurring theme: Information technology can help the nursing profession and health-care organizations survive in the increasingly competitive years ahead. And, although the use of technology can spell survival, health care institutions are not investing the kind of financial support in information systems to insure that survival. Generally, hospitals are spending 2.5% of their operating budgets on information systems, whereas other service industries are spending 7–10%.

Survival in the 1990s, said the commission, will therefore require some major reorganization in the way information is managed in the health care environment. Health care executives, recommended the commission, must therefore:

- Treat information as an asset.
- Demonstrate a strong commitment to HCIS.
- Study the benefits, strategies, and competitive advantages to be gained from HCIS.
- Establish management processes that evaluate, plan and integrate HCIS.
- Initiate effective strategic planning activities.
- Understand their role and responsibilities in collaborative efforts with computer vendors.

Vendors, on the other hand, also have specific responsibilities of their own. According to the commission, computer vendors must:

- Understand the real needs in health care by emphasizing research over product development and not simply making money.
- Reexamine their product capabilities and mix compared with needs identified by research.
- Supply what is needed rather than what is perceived as needed.
- Accelerate hardware and software integration activities.
- Support established technical protocols and standards.
- Play an increasing role in quantifying the benefits of information systems with health care organizations.

THE COMMISSION'S RECOMMENDATIONS FOR NURSING

Nursing, concluded the Commission, should be the driving force behind the integration of information systems in health care. Nursing can play a central role in not only utilizing HCIS at the bedside, but also in consulting with vendors on costs/benefits research and development of software, and with health care executives in financial planning and marketing.

HCIS can help stretch nursing resources so that patient care can be delivered in a flexible and more innovative fashion than in the past. Using HCIS can thus improve nursing productivity, nursing morale, and the long-term recruitment and retention problems which plague so many nursing departments today. Such benefits can only be realized if HCIS are reviewed as an opportunity for new horizons for nursing, and not as a threat. However, nursing must be prepared for restructuring of some nursing roles as the workplace and operations are redesigned to accommodate new technology. Although such a change may affect the FTEs in nursing, long-term benefits will be realized by the nursing profession, physicians, patients, and health-care institutions.

IMPLICATIONS FOR THE FUTURE

Through its year of research, the Secretary's Commission on Nursing has answered a critical question for the nursing profession. Information technology clearly has promising applications in health care and can indeed help the nursing shortage. However, some pertinent questions exist for the practice of nursing in the 1990s. Is the nursing profession prepared to take the quantum leap into the information age? Can nursing build information systems into standard nursing practice? Is nursing prepared to change? Above all, can nursing agree to a taxonomy and classification system for capturing nursing data?

Nursing executives interested in the concept of bedside computer terminals believe that we are now at a crossroads. The commission's findings have provided clear directions about which path to follow.

First, nursing needs to take the initiative in developing collaborative and innovative partnerships with computer vendors and other health care executives. Second, nursing can use its central role in patient care as a catalyst for convening active working groups on computer research in the health care setting. Such research will provide the essential data and documentation of operational costs, and definable benefits. Third, and perhaps most importantly, the commission's report, published in February 1989, has opened an opportunity for nursing which has far-reaching potential for helping the nursing shortage and the future of the profession as well as to provide accurate, timely and complete information essential to quality health care. We must seize this opportunity. To not do so would be a great loss for the profession.

Appendix

MECON Interviews with Hospital Personnel: Questionnaire Results

Questionnaire Results[a]

	Percent of total response					
	Hospital A		Hospital B		Hospital C	
	Pre	Post	Pre	Post	Pre	Post

Question: In what ways will the CliniCare System impact:

I. Patient care

Response:

	Pre	Post	Pre	Post	Pre	Post
1. Increased quality of care/medication errors	-0-	58.3	-0-	22	10	8
2. More accurate; less errors for documentation	38	8.3	23	-0-	7	19
3. Personalized direct care	26.5	4.1	43	4	57	27
4. More data available at one place	-0-	-0-	-0-	22	3	4
5. Less paperwork; saving in time	7	4.1	23	4	20	11
6. Vital signs and I/O more accurate	4.5	-0-	-0-	-0-	-0-	-0-
7. Others (don't know)	15	-0-	11	37	3	22
8. No impact	-0-	8.3	-0-	11	-0-	-0-
9. Taking time from patient care	-0-	16.6	-0-	22	-0-	8

II. Nursing roles (jobs)

Response:

	Pre	Post	Pre	Post	Pre	Post
1. Medical Administration/Charting easier/better decisions	-0-	4.7	-0-	-0-	33	14
2. Improve nurses productivity (more time for patient care)	58	4.7	43	25	48	21
3. Retrieval of data easier; less paperwork	8	14.2	29	-0-	-0-	-0-
4. More knowledge and better self-image	15	9.5	-0-	-0-	9	7
5. Fear of computers replacing them	4	-0-	-0-	-0-	-0-	7
6. Others (don't know)	15	4.7	28	36	3	-0-
7. More accountable	-0-	28.5	-0-	-0-	-0-	7

Questionnaire Results^a (*continued*)

	Hospital A		Hospital B		Hospital C	
	Pre	Post	Pre	Post	Pre	Post
8. More work—taking time from patient care	-0-	23.8	-0-	14	-0-	29
9. Stressed nurses—need to adjust to system	-0-	9.5	-0-	25	6	14
III. Physician role						
Response:						
1. Less satisfied with data availability/format	-0-	10.5	30	35	3	29
2. More satisfied with data availability	52	31.5	25	5	12	7
3. Less errors, centralized data, review easier	28	5.2	25	-0-	21	-0-
4. Some like, some don't; don't use, not interested	16	10.5	-0-	17	-0-	32
5. Others (don't know)	4	10.5	20	43	45	31
6. Resisting change	-0-	5.2	-0-	-0-	-0-	-0-
7. Excited/helps them	-0-	5.2	-0-	-0-	9	-0-
8. No impact	-0-	21	-0-	-0-	-0-	-0-
IV. Other						
Response:						
1. Reduce medication errors, and charging and credit problem	22	-0-	-0-	-0-	-0-	-0-
2. Pharmacy: improve recruitment, accuracy, time saving, and inventory	36	62.5	69	-0-	6	21
3. Excited because more efficient	14	-0-	-0-	-0-	-0-	-0-
4. Competitive advantage to hospital; staff will feel good	10	-0-	-0-	-0-	-0-	-0-
5. Others (nurses, PT, PT, MIS)	18	31.2	-0-	-0-	3	32
6. Patient—feel nurses' frustration	-0-	6.2	-0-	-0-	-0-	-0-
7. NR/DK, other	-0-	-0-	31	79	91	47
8. More work for pharmacy	-0-	-0-	-0-	21	-0-	-0-

Question: Which of these impacts do you feel will be most important with respect to the overall impact of the system?

Response:

1. Nursing (increase productivity)	42	37.5	25	21	46	39
2. Patient care (increased)	38	50	40	11	24	14
3. Physician	4	-0-	5	-0-	3	4
4. Equally important	4	-0-	-0-	-0-	-0-	
5. Pharmacy	-0-	12.5	20	14	-0-	4
6. Others (decrease errors, training, risk management, don't know)	12	-0-	10	54	27	39

Question: Least important

Response:

1. Physician's roles	39	64.2	30	14	24	25
2. Patient care	13	-0-	-0-	14	-0-	-0-
3. Nurses (time saving)	-0-	-0-	15	-0-	-0-	-0-
4. Competitive advantage	4	-0-	-0-	-0-	-0-	-0-
5. Pharmacy	9	7.1	-0-	-0-	-0-	-0-
6. Others	35	28.5	55	72	76	75

Question: What other benefits do you anticipate, once the full CliniCare System is installed?

Response:

1. Nurse/Pharmacy relationship improved	-0-	7.1	-0-	-0-	3	-0-
2. Less paperwork, time saving, streamline operations	32	14.2	40	7	-0-	10
3. All information for physician	19	3.5	14	-0-	-0-	-0-
4. Patient-care improvement	14	21.4	29	-0-	-0-	-0-
5. Other advantages	19	21.4	-0-	-0-	49	26
6. Don't know	11	-0-	11	46	15	2
7. Others (scary, negative feelings)	5	-0-	-0-	-0-	-0-	-0-
8. Easy to use		10.7	-0-	-0-	6	2

Questionnaire Results^a (*continued*)

	Percent of total response					
	Hospital A		Hospital B		Hospital C	
	Pre	Post	Pre	Post	Pre	Post
9. Report well organized/legible	-0-	21.4	-0-	-0-	-0-	13
10. Step toward full bar-coding/systems progress	-0-	-0-	6	11	-0-	-0-
11. More accurate medical administration and management	-0-	-0-	-0-	25	-0-	22
12. More accurate medical charting	-0-	-0-	-0-	11	-0-	-0-
13. Better record accuracy	-0-	-0-	-0-	-0-	27	19
24. Better audit trail	-0-	-0-	-0-	-0-	-0-	6

Question: How would you describe your current feelings/attitude regarding the implementation of the CliniCare terminal for point-of-care data input/retrieval?

Response:

	Hospital A		Hospital B		Hospital C	
	Pre	Post	Pre	Post	Pre	Post
1. I like the system	-0-	23	4	4	-0-	8
2. Excited/thrilled/high expectation	48	11.5	25	-0-	48	32
3. Apprehensive/concerned/frustrated	26	26.9	33	-0-	24	8
4. Concerned about trying (nervous) and physician's reaction	14	3.8	-0-	-0-	-0-	-0-
5. Others	12	-0-	-0-	21	4	25
6. Time consuming	-0-	19.2	-0-	11	-0-	-0-
7. Disappointed	-0-	3.8	-0-	8	-0-	4
8. It's the future	-0-	11.5	-0-	-0-	-0-	-0-
9. NR/DK	-0-	-0-	-0-	35	-0-	-0-

10. High expectations/welcome

	-0-	-0-	-0-	38	21	24	24
A. CliniCare will make the nurses job easier:							
Strongly disagree	-0-	11	5.8	-0-	22	-0-	9
Disagree	-0-	11	29.4	6	52	8	35
Agree	-0-	59	64.7	82	22	75	52
Strongly agree	-0-	19	-0-	12	-0-	17	4
NR	-0-	-0-	-0-	-0-	4	17	4
B. CliniCare will help capture lost charges:							
Strongly disagree	-0-	17	-0-	-0-	24	N/A	N/A
Disagree	-0-	13	22.2	19	17		
Agree	-0-	53	55.5	38	24		
Strongly agree	-0-	17	22.2	43	18		
C. CliniCare will help us keep more accurate records:							
Strongly disagree	-0-	-0-	-0-	-0-	4	-0-	5
Disagree	-0-	-0-	11.7	12	36	-0-	14
Agree	-0-	52	35.2	47	36	46	50
Strongly agree	-0-	48	52.9	41	20	54	31
NR	-0-	-0-	-0-	-0-	4	-0-	-0-
D. CliniCare will make it easier to review data at bedside:							
Strongly disagree	-0-	-0-	11.7	-0-	4	-0-	4
Disagree	-0-	18	35.2	-0-	29	-0-	-0-
Agree	-0-	48	29.4	35	38	50	70
Strongly agree	-0-	34	23.5	65	17	50	26
NR	-0-	-0-	-0-	-0-	12	-0-	-0-

Questionnaire Results[a] (continued)

	Percent of total response					
	Hospital A		Hospital B		Hospital C	
	Pre	Post	Pre	Post	Pre	Post
E. CliniCare will cause nurses to spend less time walking in the corridor:						
Strongly disagree	4	-0-	12	17	-0-	9
Disagree	40	52.9	18	46	28	22
Agree	40	47	23	17	42	55
Strongly agree	16	-0-	47	8	30	14
NR	-0-	-0-	-0-	12	-0-	-0-
F. CliniCare will enable us to provide higher quality care to our patients:						
Strongly disagree	-0-	-0-	-0-	8	-0-	5
Disagree	27	35.2	18	40	4	36
Agree	50	29.4	41	44	70	41
Strongly agree	23	35.2	41	8	26	18
G. CliniCare will make the nurse's job more interesting:						
Strongly disagree	3	-0-	-0-	8	-0-	-0-
Disagree	26	6.2	-0-	32	4	5
Agree	63	81.2	59	44	83	68
Strongly agree	8	12.5	41	8	13	27
NR	-0-	-0-	-0-	8	-0-	-0-
H. CliniCare will enable us to provide better service to physicians:						
Strongly disagree	-0-	-0-	-0-	8	-0-	-0-
Disagree	19	41.1	12	52	14	48
Agree	63	52.9	59	24	81	48
Strongly agree	18	5.8	29	-0-	5	4
NR	-0-	-0-	-0-	8	-0-	-0-

I. CliniCare will enable MD's to retrieve data faster:						
Strongly disagree	4	6.6	-0-	8	-0-	10
Disagree	8	33.3	24	32	24	65
Agree	60	46.6	41	20	67	20
Strongly agree	28	13.3	35	-0-	9	5
NR	-0-	-0-	-0-	40	-0-	-0-
J. CliniCare will improve the accuracy of medication administration:						
Strongly disagree	-0-	-0-	-0-	4	-0-	-0-
Disagree	4	5.8	6	16	4	14
Agree	22	23.5	35	44	50	32
Strongly agree	74	70.5	59	28	46	54
NR	-0-	-0-	-0-	8	-0-	-0-
K. CliniCare will improve the timeliness of medication administration:						
Strongly disagree	-0-	-0-	-0-	8	-0-	-0-
Disagree	29	11.7	35	24	4	9
Agree	29	41.1	30	40	50	41
Strongly agree	42	47	35	16	46	50
NR	-0-	-0-	-0-	12	-0-	-0-
Choose from statements below:						
a. Looks great; it will help solve a lot of our important problems	35	-0-	29	4	13	17
Midway between a and b	23	41.1	41	-0-	13	17
b. It may help solve some of our important problems	31	52.9	30	60	70	39
Midway between b and c	-0-	-0-	-0-	4	3	13
c. I doubt that it will help solve any of our important problems	11	5.8	-0-	36	-0-	13

[a]Poststudy comments: I/O accuracy, timing of vital signs, and medication administration are problems that have already been solved. The system has great potential, and we need to better adapt the organization to allow the system to help solve our problems. NR, no response.

Index